THE FAT LOSS COACH for Women

AF729794

THE FAT LOSS COACH for Women

Lose Weight
Keep it Off
Feel Incredible

Emma Storey-Gordon

Vermilion
LONDON

VERMILION

UK | USA | Canada | Ireland | Australia
India | New Zealand | South Africa

Vermilion is part of the Penguin Random House group of companies whose addresses can be found at global.penguinrandomhouse.com

Penguin Random House UK
One Embassy Gardens, 8 Viaduct Gardens, London SW11 7BW

penguin.co.uk

Penguin Random House UK

First published by Vermilion in 2026

1

Copyright © Emma Storey-Gordon 2026
Illustrations © Clarkevanmeurs 2026
The moral right of the author has been asserted.

No part of this book may be used or reproduced in any manner for the purpose of training artificial intelligence technologies or systems. In accordance with Article 4(3) of the DSM Directive 2019/790, Penguin Random House expressly reserves this work from the text and data mining exception.

Set in 11/16.2pt Kepler Std
Typeset by Six Red Marbles UK, Thetford, Norfolk

Printed and bound in Great Britain by Clays Ltd, Elcograf S.p.A.

The authorised representative in the EEA is Penguin Random House Ireland, Morrison Chambers, 32 Nassau Street, Dublin D02 YH68

A CIP catalogue record for this book is available from the British Library

ISBN 9781785046599

FSC www.fsc.org MIX Paper FSC® C018179

Penguin Random House is committed to a sustainable future for our business, our readers and our planet. This book is made from Forest Stewardship Council® certified paper.

The information in this book has been compiled as general guidance on the specific subjects addressed. It is not a substitute and not to be relied on for medical, healthcare or pharmaceutical professional advice. Please consult your GP before changing, stopping or starting any medical treatment. So far as the author is aware the information given is correct and up to date as at 26th June 2026. Practice, laws and regulations all change and the reader should obtain up-to-date professional advice on any such issues. The author and publishers disclaim, as far as the law allows, any liability arising directly or indirectly from the use or misuse of the information contained in this book.

Contents

PART 4

Your Fat-Loss Toolkit

PART 5

Hormones, Your Cycle and What Actually Changes with Age

PART 6

Making It Last

Introduction: This Is Not Another Diet Book

Let me be real with you right from the beginning. This is not a 'fresh start'. It is not a motivational reset. It is not another six-week diet plan dressed up in a different font.

This is you deciding to stop looking for quick fixes, falling for every fad and winging it when it comes to fat loss. This is you making a decision to stop letting your progress depend on motivation, the right Monday, the 'perfect time' or a version of your life that is somehow less busy than this one. That version is not coming. This is the life you have – and you get to feel your best in it.

I have spent over a decade coaching women to lose fat, build strength, stop starting over, gain control and finally break the yo-yo dieting cycle. I have answered hundreds of questions every single week for years. And the one thing I know with complete certainty is this: you are not the problem. You are exhausted and confused and have been sold nonsense your entire adult life. That stops now.

There is also something specific about the psychological experience of being a woman trying to lose weight in the world we live in – the diet culture, the shame, the large portions despite lower needs, the all-or-nothing thinking that gets baked in from an early age. The physiology matters. But what matters more is everything wrapped around it. I built my career around women because I believe women deserve an approach that takes all of this into account.

Fat loss is not complicated. It has been deliberately made to feel that way by an industry that profits from your confusion.

This book is going to fix that. By the time you finish it, you will understand exactly how fat loss works. You will be able to look at any supplement, diet trend or viral claim and know within seconds whether it is worth your attention. You will stop falling for things that were never going to work. And you will have the tools to help you lose fat and keep it off for the rest of your life, not just the next six weeks.

That is the promise. Let me tell you why I can keep it.

Why Listen to Me

This is the first question you should always be asking when taking advice generally. Growing up, I had energy, drive and a genuine desire to make an impact on the world. What I lacked was a clear sense of where to target it. Except sport. Sport I always understood. So I followed that thread and studied Sport Science at the University of Edinburgh.

For most of my degree, I was fine. Not passionate, just fine. Then, in my final year, I took a module on exercise and health. Learning about the impact of exercise on cardiovascular disease, type 2 diabetes and certain cancers genuinely blew my mind. That was the first time I thought: this actually matters. This is life-changing.

After university, I worked in research. I measured plaque in arteries, tested insulin sensitivity and looked at blood markers of inflammation. Later, I joined projects using exercise to help breast cancer survivors. It was fascinating, but it was also painfully slow. I am naturally very impatient – I wanted to help people *now*, not in five years when a paper finally gets published. So I left academia and went all in on coaching.

Very quickly, I realised something important: fat loss is not about the perfect diet or the optimal workout plan; it is about behaviour, mindset and consistency. A good coach can write you a plan. A great coach can get you to stick to it. That is what I became obsessed with.

I have now coached tens of thousands of women through every possible variation of this. High-flying career women, busy mothers, women going through menopause, women who have been dieting since their teens and feel like they have tried everything; women who are successful in every other area of their lives but somehow cannot crack this one. I have seen patterns that no textbook will ever teach you. I've watched women spend years cycling through protocols that were never going to work, blaming themselves when they didn't. I've watched the supplement industry get richer while women get more anxious about their cortisol levels. I've watched social media turn genuinely interesting nutrition science into a horror story designed to make women afraid of carbohydrates and dependent on monitoring devices they don't need. I've watched 'empowerment' get used as a sales tool so successfully that the women being sold to can't even see it happening. It made me angry. It still does. That anger turned out to be great motivation and is where this book came from.

I know what actually works and what people say works but does not. I understand why smart, disciplined women keep falling for the same traps – and, most importantly, how to get out of them for good. I have also built one of the largest fitness communities in the UK, with tens of thousands of people reading and listening every week. I tell you this not to impress you but to say: I have stress-tested the ideas in this book at scale. They work. And if you want to lose fat and keep it off for life, you are in the right place.

One more thing: in the age of the influencer, where anyone with a large following is treated as an authority, please be sceptical of everything. If a claim sounds too good to be true, it usually is – and it's usually someone trying to sell you something. Always ask for evidence. Always ask how something works. If someone cannot explain why their approach works beyond 'it worked for me' or 'my clients love it', that is not good enough.

This is the standard I hold myself to. If I make a claim in this book, I have shown my workings. If I recommend something, I have explained why, with evidence, not just because it worked for a client or because I believe it to be true. That is the bar, and it should be the bar for everyone giving advice on your health.

What This Book Is and Is Not

This is not a meal plan. I am not going to tell you what to eat for breakfast on a Tuesday. Instead, this book gives you the understanding to make your own informed decisions, for the rest of your life. The science of fat loss is simple, and you will learn it in the first chapter. The rest of the book is about why it is hard to apply, what gets in the way, the lies and half-truths you've been told that leave so many of us confused and overwhelmed, and the practical tools that allow you to make this the last time you ever need to lose fat. Because this time, you will keep it off.

The book is structured in six parts. Part 1 covers the science because before we can change anything, we need to understand how fat loss actually works and why it feels so complicated. We'll also get practical right from the start as, in this section, I'll also show you how to set up your fat-loss calories in a way that actually works. This knowledge will give you the power to lose fat without losing your mind, and you will never be conned again by fad diets and supplements. Before you can move forward with confidence, though, we also need to unpack the myths, misinformation and industry noise that may have been holding you back. So, Part 2 – The Bullsh*t Files – gives you the lowdown on the supplement and wellness industry, and the people making money from your confusion. Part 3 is all about the simple mindset shifts that will support you in your journey and Part 4 is where we connect everything you have learned into a set of practical, adaptable tools – from how to manage hunger, sleep and exercise to dealing with the moments when you're tempted to say 'f*ck it'. These aren't strict 'rules' or a prescriptive system, but principles you can adapt depending on where you are and what your life looks like right now. Part 5 covers hormones, your menstrual cycle, menopause and ageing, so you can use the tools to work *with* your physiology, not against it, whatever stage of life you're in. Finally, Part 6 is all about making fat loss last.

Try to read the book from the beginning all the way through

if you can, as each part builds on the one before it, helping you cut through the noise, truly understand your body and approach fat loss in a way that finally feels sustainable. Of course, if a particular chapter title is calling your name, do go there first. This is your book, so read it in the way that feels right for you.

One Thing Before We Start

I want to take the shame out of body fat right from the beginning: fat is something you have, it is not something you are.

Biologically, body fat is stored energy. That is it. It does not define you, it does not make you lazy and it does not make you a bad person. There are many reasons why some people store more fat than others: genetics, hormones, environment, life stress – and all of it is changeable.

The truth is, we live in an environment where being overweight is the norm. If you're not actively being conscious about staying lean then you will most likely gain weight, because of the combination of our human drive to eat and the abundance of extremely tasty food that tempts us at every turn.

There is so much shame around storing extra energy (body fat) – but shame does not create lasting change. It creates restriction, usually followed by bingeing, followed by more shame. I have seen this cycle destroy years of progress for women who were doing almost everything right. As you work through these pages, treat yourself like someone you want to win. Support yourself the way you would someone you love. You wouldn't try to shame them into change – you already know that wouldn't work – so don't do the same to yourself.

A Note on How I Coach

My approach is built on a core principle: imperfect action, consistently applied, beats a perfect plan you can only manage on perfect days. You can go over your calories every single day, never finish a full workout and miss your step target most of the week and still lose fat. You can be far from perfect and still get results. What you cannot do is quit every time something goes wrong and expect things to change.

If this resonates with you, this time will be different, not because of me or the information in this book. But because *you* are different. Because you are deciding, right now, to stop looking for excuses and start looking for solutions.

'I don't quit. I just adjust and keep going.'

That is the only rule you need. If you keep going, keep adjusting and stop treating every slip as a reason to give up, this will be the last time you need to start.

I am also keen on making things as easy and efficient as possible. The best way to lose fat is to make it simple and apply the principles you learn here in a way that works for you and your life. The scientific understanding of fat loss will allow you to do this. You will soon see that most people have been making fat loss way harder and more complicated than it needs to be.

Ready? Let's go.

A note on readership: while this book is written for women, the science of fat loss discussed here applies to anyone. If you are reading this and do not identify as a woman, the principles throughout are just as relevant to you – the female-specific chapters simply provide additional context for readers who navigate the societal, cultural, hormonal and physiological realities described there.

PART 1

CRACKING THE CODE

Part 1 is your foundation. In the next chapters, you will learn the science of how fat loss happens, why it is genuinely harder for women to lose weight compared to men (and why that is not an excuse), why the process feels so complicated when the science itself is simple, and how to track your progress and work out your own calorie needs so you can finally get results that last.

Everything that comes after this part builds on what you learn here. Read it carefully, even if some of it feels familiar. These details matter.

Chapter 1

The Science of Fat Loss

My aim for this chapter is for you to understand how fat loss actually happens, what people tend to get wrong and, most importantly, for you to feel empowered to apply this knowledge in a way that works for you.

Understanding fat loss starts with understanding what fat actually is.

The Energy Balance Equation

Body fat is your body's long-term energy storage system. When you take in more energy than you use, the excess is stored, primarily as fat. When you use more energy than you take in, your body dips into those stores to make up the shortfall – this is called a 'calorie deficit'. That is the whole mechanism. Everything else – every diet, every protocol, every approach you have ever tried – is just a different way of influencing one or both sides of this energy balance equation. (We'll look at how to calculate your own calorie deficit in Chapter 5.)

The energy you take in is straightforward: it is the food and drink you consume. There are a few nuances around how much of the food you take in is digested and utilised, but, put simply, it's the food and drink you consume.

Your energy expenditure is slightly more interesting, because it has four components, and the one most people focus on – exercise – is actually the smallest:

1. **Your BMR, or basal metabolic rate,** is the energy your body uses just to keep you alive: breathing, your heartbeat, maintaining your organs, keeping your temperature stable. This accounts for roughly 60–70 per cent of your total daily energy expenditure. It is mostly determined by your body size and muscle mass.
2. **NEAT stands for non-exercise activity thermogenesis.** This is all the movement you do that is not formal exercise: walking to your car, doing the washing-up, fidgeting, gesticulating when you talk. It accounts for around 15–20 per cent of your energy out and, critically, it is the most variable component. Two people with similar bodies can differ by up to 2,000 calories a day in NEAT. It is also the first thing your body unconsciously reduces when you are in a calorie deficit.
3. **EAT is exercise activity thermogenesis.** This is your actual workouts and accounts for roughly 5 per cent of your total energy out – less than most people think. Exercise is incredibly important for health, body composition and maintaining your results, but it is not a reliable way to create a large calorie deficit on its own. Athletes and those who train for endurance events will often find their contribution is significantly higher,

but for most people, the gym alone will not move the needle without dietary changes.

4. **TEF is the thermic effect of food.** This is the energy your body uses to digest what you eat and accounts for around 10 per cent of your energy expenditure.

The word 'fat' carries so many negative connotations but, as you now understand, it simply means someone has taken in more energy than they have used over time. When that happens, your body does exactly what it was designed to do – it stores the excess energy as fat tissue, holding it in reserve for a time when food might be scarce. That is not a malfunction. That is a survival system that kept our ancestors alive.

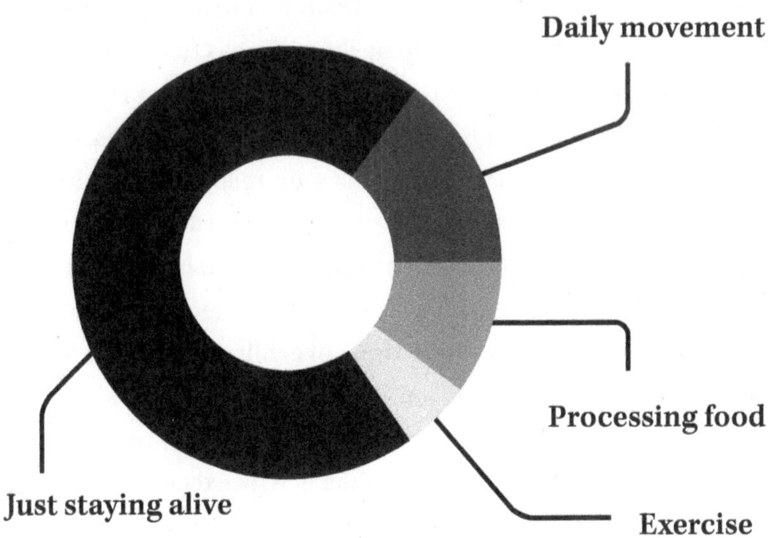

Calories you burn in a day

The problem is that we are now living in an environment for which our biology was never built. Food is abundant, heavily engineered to override fullness signals, and available at every turn. We are more sedentary than any generation before us. We are more stressed, more sleep-deprived and more time-poor. These factors push the body towards storing more and burning less. It is not a character flaw. It is not laziness.

That said, excess body fat is not just stored energy with no consequences. And just because it's not your fault, that doesn't mean it's not your responsibility. Too much fat is a health issue. When fat cells become overfilled, they start to malfunction. Instead of simply storing energy, they release inflammatory signals that spread through the body and begin to interfere with the way cells normally work. One of the key casualties of this is something known as 'insulin sensitivity'. Normally, insulin – a hormone produced by the pancreas to regulate blood sugar – acts like a key that unlocks your cells so they can absorb glucose from the blood, but these inflammatory signals make the lock harder to turn. Your cells stop responding to insulin properly, your pancreas has to produce more and more of it to compensate, and blood glucose begins to rise. This is called 'insulin resistance', and it is the primary mechanism behind type 2 diabetes. At the same time, overfilled fat cells generate 'oxidative stress' – a build-up of damaging molecules that put pressure on your metabolism at a cellular level, a process sometimes called 'metabolic stress'. This is why excess fat, particularly around the abdomen where it sits closest to your vital organs, is so strongly associated with type 2 diabetes and cardiovascular disease.

Your Personal Fat Threshold

One thing worth knowing is that not everyone stores fat in the same way. Everyone has what researchers call a 'personal fat threshold': the point at which your fat cells are full and fat starts being stored in places it should not be, like your liver and muscle tissue. This is where the metabolic problems described above begin.

Some people are genetically able to carry a significant amount of body fat before reaching this threshold. Others hit it at a lower body weight and develop metabolic issues while still appearing relatively lean – things like elevated blood glucose, high triglycerides, raised blood pressure, poor insulin sensitivity or early-stage fatty liver disease. This is why you genuinely cannot judge someone's health by how they look. A person can be slim and metabolically unwell, and a person can carry more fat than the charts say they should while remaining metabolically healthy. Where you store your body fat, not just how much, is important.

The good news is that understanding the science of body fat means you can control it, change it and remove the unnecessary guilt around it.

Where Fat Goes When You Lose It

Have you ever wondered where fat actually goes when you lose it? Most people say they sweat it out. Or burn it off. Or, my personal favourite, that it turns into muscle. None of those are correct. The answer is genuinely fascinating and also a bit bizarre: you breathe it out.

Fat is broken down inside your cells. It is then stored in the body in the form of triglycerides – think of them as your body's preferred packaging for long-term energy, made up of three fatty acid chains (the actual fuel) attached to a small backbone molecule called glycerol. When you are in a calorie deficit and your body needs to draw on its fat stores, fatty acids and glycerol are released into the bloodstream. The fatty acids are then transported into your mitochondria – the structures inside your cells responsible for producing energy – where they are oxidised, meaning they react with oxygen and are systematically dismantled. The glycerol, meanwhile, heads to the liver to be converted into glucose. The end products of this entire process are carbon dioxide and water. The majority of the fat you lose leaves your body through your lungs as CO_2. You do not melt fat. You do not sweat it out. You exhale it.

This was confirmed by a 2014 study published in *The BMJ*, which tracked exactly where the atoms in fat molecules go during weight loss. The researchers found that when you lose 10kg of fat, roughly 8.4kg of it is exhaled as carbon dioxide. The rest leaves as water, through urine, sweat and breath. Every breath you take out is, in a tiny way, fat loss in action.

The science of fat loss can be learned in a single chapter. The rest of this book is about everything the industry has piled on top of it, and how to cut through all of it.

You now know the science. Everything that follows is about making it work in your actual life.

KEY POINTS

- Fat is simply stored energy, not a character flaw or a weakness.
- NEAT, your non-exercise daily movement, contributes far more to your energy expenditure than your gym sessions. Your step count matters.
- When you lose fat, you exhale most of it as carbon dioxide. You breathe it out.

Chapter 2

Why Fat Loss Is Harder for Women (and Why That's Not an Excuse)

Now that you understand how fat loss actually works at a biological level, it is time to look at something that is rarely talked about: why this process is genuinely harder for women and exactly where that difficulty comes from.

A client came to me a few years ago absolutely convinced that something was wrong with her body. She had been eating less than her husband for years. She trained more than him. She was more consistent, more disciplined, more careful with everything she put in her mouth. And he was losing weight, and she was not. She was not imagining it. It was genuinely harder for her, but not for the reasons she thought. No broken metabolism. No rare hormonal condition. No mysterious physiological defect. Just the ordinary, infuriating reality of being a woman trying to lose fat in a world that has mostly been designed around male bodies.

I want to be clear before we go any further: this chapter is not about using the fact that you are a woman as an excuse. Instead, I'm going to give you an accurate map so you understand why fat loss is genuinely harder for you – and can maybe give yourself some grace and credit for doing hard things!

The Great Female-Specific Con

Before we get into what is actually different about male and female fat loss, I want to address what is not.

On a physiological level, there are not many meaningful differences between men and women when it comes to losing fat or building muscle. The confusion comes from the fact that women are obviously different to men physically, hormonally and biologically. But that does not mean the science of energy storage, how we use it or what builds muscle is fundamentally different.

Marketers thrive on telling you otherwise. They love the idea that women need a completely different approach because it lets them sell you something unique, something with a premium price tag and an empowerment narrative wrapped around it. It's the classic 'pink tax' – the tendency for products or, in this case, diets or coaching programmes marketed to women to cost more than when marketed to men.

There is a dangerous trend on social media where brands and influencers promote female-specific programmes as though the basic rules of physiology do not apply to women. This misinformation confuses women and makes them feel like they are doing something wrong. It leads to overcomplicating the process to the point where many women take no action at all. That is what makes it so dangerous, as it is taking years of healthy life span from women who are so worried about doing the wrong thing that they end up doing nothing.

I talk to women every week who have stopped exercising because they were told that high-intensity interval training (HIIT) is bad for them. Who do not lift weights because someone told them they would get bulky. Who eat no carbs after 6pm because an influencer insisted it causes fat gain. It is no wonder so many women are scared to do anything in case it is the wrong thing. And then there are the people adamantly claiming that something is the secret to fat loss while others are claiming it is the cause of fat gain. A classic example of this is fasting. Some will claim that fasting is the only way to lose fat because it forces your body into 'fat-burning mode'. Others claim that fasting puts your body into starvation mode and you will store more calories, seemingly from nowhere.

You can see why it's confusing!

What Is Actually Different

As you now know, the fundamentals of fat loss are the same for everyone – it all comes down to the energy balance equation we looked at in the previous chapter. But despite the fundamentals being identical, it is genuinely harder for women, just not for the reasons you are usually told.

Here is what is actually going on.

Body size and calorie needs

Women generally have less lean body mass and smaller bodies than men. This means a lower resting metabolic rate, which is the number of calories your body burns just to keep you alive.

This is not actually a sex difference. It is a body size difference. If a woman had the same height, weight and muscle mass as a man, their metabolic rates would be very similar. It just happens that most women are, on average, smaller, which means most women need fewer calories.

And fewer calories means less room for error. If a man burns 3,000 calories a day, a 20 per cent deficit is 600 calories. If a woman burns 2,000, that same 20 per cent is only 400 calories. It is much easier to accidentally eat back a 400-calorie deficit through small inaccuracies in tracking or slightly larger portions than you intended (I will cover the inaccuracy in calorie tracking and how to ensure you don't fall outside of your deficit in Chapter 5).

This is why you might feel like you are in a deficit but are still not losing weight. Tracking calories is very hard to do accurately and, with a smaller margin for error, it's much easier for these inaccuracies to add up and result in a lack of fat loss despite your best efforts. And that can be really demotivating. This often leads to us turning to more extreme approaches, and it makes sense – why would you stick to something that isn't working?

Hormones and the menstrual cycle

The hormones oestrogen and progesterone fluctuate throughout the month, affecting appetite, cravings, water retention and mood. For many women, the week before their period brings the sharpest drop in motivation and the biggest increase in hunger.

This is certainly true for me. I usually want to quit my job and eat an entire cake the week before my period. I also get hormonal migraines that mean lying in a dark room is the only option. Being honest about this matters because it is so common and yet so rarely talked about.

The impact on dietary adherence – your ability to stick to your diet – during those few days a month is real. We will cover the menstrual cycle in detail in Chapter 23, including what actually helps.

The menopause transition

As oestrogen declines as we age, many women experience symptoms that make fat loss significantly harder: poor sleep, increased anxiety and a shift in where fat is stored, often towards the stomach. The way fat loss works does not change during perimenopause or post-menopause, but the symptoms can make the process much more difficult. If you are in this life stage, the good news is that Chapter 24 is dedicated to managing this.

Psychological and societal pressure

Women are more heavily targeted by the weight-loss industry than men. A higher percentage of women than men attempt to lose weight – 56.4 per cent versus 41.7 per cent – despite broadly similar obesity rates between the sexes. When it comes to weight-loss supplements specifically, women use them at more than double the rate of men. The pressure to be lean sits more heavily on women, and many women link their body image more directly to their self-worth in a way that men often do not. Research has found that 70 per cent of women rate their current figure as larger than their ideal, compared to 33 per cent of men.

This is not an accident of nature. It is the result of decades of deliberate cultural messaging about what a woman's body should look like. The ideal of thinness, launched by the fashion industry in the 1960s, became and remains the idealised standard of beauty in Western culture and its influence falls disproportionately on women. Research consistently shows that in Western societies, beauty is more essential to the feminine gender role than the masculine one, and that body size is a more relevant factor for women's self-worth than for men's. Women are shown a narrower, more prescriptive ideal – thin, toned, young – repeated back at them through media, advertising and social comparison, from childhood onwards, whereas men's body ideals are more varied and more forgiving. The result is a market of women who have been conditioned to feel perpetually not quite right in their own skin. And where there is that feeling, there is an industry ready to sell you the solution.

Women also still carry the majority of household labour and caregiving. A 2024 study from the University of Bath and the University of Melbourne found that mothers take on 71 per cent of all household mental load tasks – the scheduling, planning and organising that keeps family life running; 60 per cent more than fathers. That is before you factor in the physical tasks: cooking, cleaning, childcare. That kind of invisible labour requires enormous time and energy, and it rarely appears on anyone's to-do list because it never stops. When you are exhausted from looking after everyone else, time for yourself and your own goals is almost always the first thing to disappear.

What This Means in Practice

Fat loss is harder for women for real, legitimate reasons. On top of that, we live in an environment where food is in abundance and portion sizes are way beyond our needs. Therefore, if you want results, you need to accept the reality we live in and choose to change anyway. It might not be fair, but you get to decide whether you use these challenges as reasons not to try or whether you accept the constraints and decide you are still going to get results. Because as much as it is hard to stay lean in the world we live in, it's certainly not impossible and it's absolutely worth it to feel your best.

The fundamental science of fat loss is the same for men and women. The physiology of energy storage and muscle building does not operate differently based on sex. Marketing that tells you otherwise is selling you something (and probably adding a pink tax to it!). You do not need a special female diet. You do not need to adjust your food around your menstrual cycle or avoid particular exercises at certain times of the month. Instead, you need an approach that accounts for the realities of female physiology, that is honest about the extra challenges and that gives you the tools to work with your body rather than against it. That is exactly what this book does.

Now that you understand the real differences, let us look at why fat loss feels so complicated, and what to do about it.

KEY POINTS

- Women generally need fewer calories than men not because of their sex, but because of their size. And lower calorie needs means a smaller margin for tracking error – that margin is where many women unknowingly lose their deficit.
- Hormonal fluctuations across the menstrual cycle – particularly the week before your period – affect appetite, cravings, water retention and mood. This makes adherence genuinely harder at certain points in the month.
- Menopause symptoms including poor sleep, increased hunger and anxiety, low mood and motivation, and shifts in fat distribution make the process harder. The mechanism of fat loss does not change, but the conditions you are working in do.
- Women carry a disproportionate share of domestic labour and caregiving. You need a plan that realistically fits around your life.
- Society places enormous pressure on women to look a certain way – and that pressure often drives women to pursue fat loss from a place of shame rather than health. Sustainable fat loss requires a relationship with food and your body that diet culture actively works against.
- You do not need a special female diet. You need an approach that is realistic about the challenges and works with your body and your life, not against it.

Chapter 3

Why Fat Loss Feels So Complicated

'Lose ten pounds in a month on keto.' That is the kind of headline that gets a million views. Sensible calorie deficit, adequate protein, daily movement and decent sleep – all the key components of fat loss that this book will explain – those things do not go viral and they do not sell a programme, diet or supplement.

Extremes sell. Balance is boring. And an entire industry has been built on making fat loss feel complicated, overwhelming and so full of contradictions that you feel like you're missing out on some secret that has been eluding you all this time. In this chapter, we'll cut through the bullsh*t and look at how people are making a lot of money from selling you programmes, supplements and new approaches to solve problems that do not exist – and, importantly, what actually works.

Why Social Media Makes Things Worse

On social media, everyone has a voice, and those voices are weighted equally regardless of qualifications. A large following is perceived as credibility. In reality, the biggest accounts often grow through extreme, attention-grabbing messaging rather than evidence-based advice.

I would even argue that the bigger the following, the more sceptical you should be. Nuance does not go viral. Saying 'it depends' does not get shares. But saying 'cut out all carbs and you will lose ten pounds this month' does. Saying 'this supplement completely changed my life' also does.

Credentials don't automatically fix this either. Someone can have impressive qualifications and still be significantly outside their area of expertise when it comes to fat loss. Having a background in one area of health is extraordinarily valuable. It is not, however, the same as having expertise in exercise science, sports nutrition or fat-loss coaching. These are different disciplines. Yet a set of credentials can lend credibility to claims that the evidence does not support.

Be especially careful of medical professionals who describe the mainstream advice as corrupt, biased or designed only for men. Sometimes, that critique has merit. Often, it is a way of delegitimising the tools, peer review, randomised controlled trials or meta-analyses that would allow you to scrutinise their own claims.

The Best Diet is the One You Can Stick to

The reason fat loss seems so full of contradictions is that people focus on the method rather than the mechanism. The reality is that every diet that has ever worked has worked for the same reason. The debates about carbs versus fat, fasting versus eating six meals a day, keto versus flexible dieting . . . these are not debates about whether the fundamental science works. They are debates about which method makes it easier for a particular person to sustain a calorie deficit. That is all. There is a famous analogy in physics: all roads lead to Rome. In fat loss, all roads lead to a calorie deficit. The road you choose should be the one you can actually walk.

A landmark meta-analysis published in *JAMA* in 2014 compared popular diets, including low-carb, low-fat, Mediterranean and others. The researchers found that after 12 months, the differences in weight loss between the diets were modest and largely insignificant. What predicted success was not the diet type. It was adherence to whatever diet the person had chosen.

Read that again: the best diet is the one you can stick to. This is either the most liberating thing you will read in this book or, if you were hoping for a more complicated answer, possibly the most disappointing. There is no secret. There is no shortcut. There is the energy balance equation we looked at in Chapter 1, and then there is everything else people have built around it to make it seem more complex, more proprietary and more worth selling.

Low-carb works. Fasting works. Tracking calories works. A Mediterranean diet works. They all work for exactly the same reason.

This is why the best diet for fat loss is the one you can actually stick to, consistently, without feeling completely miserable. I personally prefer a lower-carb approach when I want to lose fat because I find it keeps me full. Others would hate that. I have got into the best shape of my life using completely different methods at different times. I have got lean while intermittent fasting, I have got lean while reducing carbs and I have got lean using the 3:1 method (my preferred approach which I will share with you later). All three times, the mechanism was that I created a sustained calorie deficit. You would not be able to look at me and tell the difference between the three approaches. The outcome was the same because the principle was the same.

We'll be fully unpicking the misinformation that abounds in the diet and fitness industry in Part 2, but, for now, next time you hear a new fat-loss claim, ask yourself: does this help me create a calorie deficit? If yes, it might work. Then, you need to consider whether it is an enjoyable way for you to create a deficit. For example, if you are someone who doesn't mind missing breakfast and pushing your first meal a little later and you're not prone to overeating, intermittent fasting might be for you. Or you might think that it sounds awful. You might absolutely love carbs, in which case a low-carb diet is unlikely to be a good option for you. You might instead prefer to track your calories.

Knowledge is power. Understanding how fat loss works gives you control, confidence and results that last, because you actually understand how you achieved them.

The End-Point Fallacy

Most diets fail because they were never designed to work long term. They are sold as six- to eight-week programmes with a defined end point because that is easier to market. You can put a before and after photo on it. You can count down to it. And you can sell it again and again.

However, if you want to keep your results, you need to keep

the behaviours that created them – forever. The numbers on the scales may shift a little over time, but the fundamentals do not change. You cannot reach the end of a six-week diet, go back to everything you were doing before and expect the results to stay.

Think of it like this: if you get your hedge trimmed in the garden, it will look good for a few weeks. But if you want it to stay neat, you need to keep trimming it. Your body works in exactly the same way.

Health and fitness are not things you ever finish. You are never permanently 'done' taking care of your body, just as you are never permanently done trimming your hedge if you want it to remain neat. This is not a depressing thought. It is actually a freeing one. Because it means you do not need to be perfect. You just need to be consistent enough, over time, to build a life that supports the body you want.

Teaching people what to do is the easy part. The real art of coaching is helping people stick to what they already know they need to do. Losing fat and keeping it off is as much about psychology as it is about nutrition. On paper, fat loss is an energy deficit. In practice, it requires managing emotions, cravings, a social life, a busy household and sometimes years of ingrained self-sabotage.

This is why Part 3 is about the practical tools you need to help you apply the science consistently. The knowledge alone is not enough. If it were, everyone who had ever read a diet book would be lean.

The industry profits from your confusion.
The science is simple. You are not broken. You are just overcomplicating it.

KEY POINTS

- The confusion around fat loss is largely manufactured. An entire industry profits from making you feel like you are missing a secret. You are not.
- The most extreme claims get the most shares – and that is exactly why you should be most sceptical of them.
- A large social media following is not the same as credibility and medical qualifications in one discipline do not confer expertise in another. A doctor with a social media platform is not automatically an authority on fat loss, exercise science or sports nutrition.
- Every diet that has ever worked has worked by creating a calorie deficit. This is why so many different diets 'work'.
- The best diet is the one you can actually stick to.
- Most diets are designed with an end point because that is easier to sell. But keeping your results requires keeping the behaviours that created them. There is no finish line. You have to take care of your body for life.

Chapter 4

What the Scales Are Actually Measuring

With the science of fat loss clear and the manufactured confusion dismantled, there is one more trap to address: the weighing scales. How you read and respond to your weight data will make or break your consistency – and most people are doing it wrong.

It is criminal how many diets are derailed by placing too much importance on the number shown on the scales. More specifically, by a fundamental misunderstanding of what that number actually means. One of the most heartbreaking things for me as a fat-loss coach is seeing clients put in so much work, do all the right things, make progress and then blow it all up because the scales don't show what they were expecting. Without being dramatic, in my experience, misinterpretation of the scales ruins more otherwise successful diets for women than any other single factor.

Your scale weight is not a measure of your body fat. It is a measure of your total mass at that moment in time: fat, muscle, bone, water, the contents of your digestive system, and everything else your body contains. It weighs all of it. It cannot distinguish between them.

Think logically for a second. Unless you are a weight-class athlete, nobody cares what you weigh. You do not walk around with your weight written on your forehead. What matters is how you feel, how you perform and how you look for yourself, not anyone else. When you focus on those things, the weight takes care of itself. But when you let one number on one morning determine your entire emotional state, you hand over an enormous amount of power to something that is not measuring the right thing. It is insane.

I often play out a scenario where you need to explain the ridiculousness of the scale weight and the control it has over women to an alien. The aliens would think we were mad: *You are letting a number dictate your day? Your mood? Your self-worth? Let me get this straight: a number that doesn't even measure what you think it does? A number that fluctuates every day and constantly throughout the day for reasons that have nothing to do with the outcome you care about – fat gain or loss? Interesting.* Aren't humans interesting!

Why the Number Moves (and It Has Nothing to Do with Fat)

There are dozens of things that impact your scale weight that have absolutely nothing to do with body fat. Most are related to water retention or what I will politely call gut content: literally how much food and waste is currently inside you.

Salt intake moves it. High sodium causes your body to retain water. A Chinese takeaway the night before can add a kilogram or more to your morning weight with zero fat gained.

Sleep has an impact. Poor sleep increases inflammation and water retention.

Travel has an effect. Being on a long flight, eating airport and plane food with a high salt content, disrupted sleep . . . all of it shows up on the scales.

Exercise moves it. A hard training session causes micro-damage to muscle tissue, which your body responds to with inflammation and fluid. You can weigh more after a good workout than before it.

And your bathroom habits move it. This one is obvious but often overlooked.

Hormones have an impact too (more on this shortly).

There is one line I like to remind clients of: if you gain weight overnight, it is not body fat. To actually gain one pound of body fat, you need to consume approximately 3,500 calories above your maintenance needs. Your maintenance level is simply the number of calories your body needs in a day to stay exactly as it is – not gaining, not losing, just ticking over (this is also known as your total daily energy expenditure, or TDEE). It accounts for everything: your resting metabolism, your movement and your digestion. When you eat above that number consistently over time, the surplus gets stored as fat. When you eat below it, your body draws on fat stores to make up the shortfall. The 3,500 figure refers to how far above that maintenance level you would need to eat to store one additional pound of fat.

So, if the scales say you put on three pounds overnight, you would have needed to eat a surplus of over 10,000 calories above your maintenance the previous day. Unless you ate the entire contents of your fridge and chased it with a bottle of oil, that did not happen. It is water. It is food volume. It is not fat. Now, if you gain weight consistently over weeks, it most likely is body fat, but short-term fluctuations on the scales do not represent changes in body composition.

You will have weeks where you gain weight and lose fat simultaneously. If you do not accept this, you will think a plan is not working and you will quit. It is one of the most important things I can tell you because if you quit every time the scales go up you will NEVER get results.

The Menstrual Cycle and the Scales

I cannot talk about fluctuations on the scales without talking about your menstrual cycle too. For women, the monthly hormonal shifts make scale fluctuations bigger and more emotionally loaded than they already are.

In the week before your period, progesterone can cause significant water retention. You can wake up two or three pounds heavier overnight while being in a genuine calorie deficit. In fact, it is very common to be losing fat in the days before your period while the scales go up. If you do not understand this, it looks like failure. But it's not.

The general pattern most women experience looks like this: in the first two weeks after their period the scales tend to cooperate, weight is lower and energy is higher. Around ovulation, there is a small spike. In the week before their period, the scales go up, hunger increases, mood drops and body image takes a hit. Then their period arrives, they drop the water, and suddenly the scales go back down.

If you don't know what to expect, you're very likely to give up even though you are losing weight. For example: I usually gain 3lb the week before my period. If I was in a 500-calorie-a-day deficit I could expect to lose about 1lb a week of fat. This means that the week before my period it is likely I will weigh 2lb more but still have lost fat. This causes a lot of women to give up or drop calories. It's really hard to be rational and logical when your mood is low, body image is impacted, hunger and cravings are higher and irritability is peaking (I speak for myself here!), but going in with this knowledge sets you up well. Hold tight because you will look back a week later and be proud you did.

How to Use the Scales Without Them Using You

People tend to respond to the scales going up in one of two ways:

1. They quit. This is the woman who gives up on her diet because she has not lost weight after three days. Three days. Fat loss is measured in weeks, not days, and the scales on day three are telling you nothing about whether your approach is working.
2. They slash their calories. This is the woman who gains a pound over the weekend, panics and immediately drops her calories to something she cannot sustain. This almost never results in better fat loss. It usually results in a miserable week followed by a binge that eliminates any deficit she created.

Both of these patterns have the same cause: too much emotional weight placed on the scales.

Before you panic, I am not going to tell you to throw away the scales. Weight data is useful. But there is a right way and a wrong way to use them.

If you do decide to weigh yourself, weigh yourself consistently, at the same time, under the same conditions, in the morning after you've used the bathroom and before food. If you weigh yourself at random times, you are comparing incomparable numbers and making an inaccurate measurement even less accurate.

Use your lowest weight from the week and compare week on week. A trend across four to six weeks tells you something real. A single Tuesday morning reading tells you almost nothing. Interestingly, sometimes having people weigh themselves daily actually improves their relationship with the scales because they see how much the numbers fluctuate even when they haven't changed their diet. When you know you're in a deficit but you still see the scales go up and down day to day and you've stuck to it long enough to know that when you are consistent they trend down, you start to get your head around the daily fluctuations without freaking out or it impacting your mood or behaviours.

It's also important to track other things alongside your weight, such as:

- How your clothes fit.
- Your measurements – specifically your waist circumference, which is a strong indication of metabolic health.
- How you feel.
- Your strength in the gym.
- Your energy levels.

These are all measures of progress that the scales cannot capture.

And if the scales are making you miserable, consistently ruining your day or causing you to make impulsive decisions to eat more or eat less, consider whether they are actually helping you. For some of my clients, removing the scales entirely leads to better results because they stop the emotional spiral and stay consistent with the behaviours. The goal is fat loss. The scales are just one tool to measure it. Removing the scales and focusing on your actions and letting the outcome take care of itself is often a much more positive and effective approach.

Remember: the scales are a data point. Not a verdict on your effort. Not a measure of your worth. Not a conclusive measure of your progress and certainly not a reason to quit.

Your scale weight is a piece of useful data when used in context and understood correctly. Treat it accordingly.

KEY POINTS

- Your scale weight is your total body mass at that moment: fat, muscle, water, bone and gut content. It cannot tell you how much fat you have lost.
- Weight can fluctuate by several pounds in a single day due to water retention, salt intake, stress, sleep, exercise and your digestive system. None of this is body fat.
- To gain one pound of fat, you need a 3,500-calorie surplus. If the scale goes up three pounds overnight, it is water. Not fat.
- Before your period, progesterone causes significant water retention. You can be in a genuine calorie deficit and still see the scales rise. This is very common and very normal.
- Use the lowest weight from the week and compare your weight week on week, not day to day.

- Track multiple measures of progress, not just scale weight.
- If the scales are consistently making you spiral, it is okay to step back from daily weigh-ins. Better behaviour and worse data is often a better trade-off than worse behaviour and more data.

Chapter 5

Setting Up Your Fat-Loss Calories in a Way That Actually Works

You understand the science of fat loss, can see through the industry noise and now know that in order to lose fat you need to be in a calorie deficit. So, before we go any further, you need to learn how to calculate your personal deficit and free yourself from all-or-nothing thinking. Once you have that foundation, everything else will click into place.

Setting Your Fat-Loss Calories

As a reminder, a calorie deficit simply means using more energy than you take in so your body is forced to use its own energy – body fat – for fuel. To work out your own personal calorie deficit, you first need to find out your maintenance calories or total daily energy expenditure (TDEE) – this is simply the number of calories that keep your weight stable over time.

The most reliable way to find this is to track your calorie intake for two to three weeks while your weight is stable – that number is your maintenance. However, though this might be the most reliable way, it's also very time-consuming and is dependent on your ability to track accurately. As you'll come to see, not many people have this ability – myself included – and it gets boring pretty fast! So, a more practical way to estimate your maintenance is to use an online TDEE calculator, which takes your height, weight, age and a rough activity level, and applies a formula to estimate your needs. These are widely available and free.

It is worth being honest about what these numbers are, though: they are educated guesses. The formulas are built from population averages, which means they can be meaningfully off for any individual. Your actual TDEE depends on your precise muscle mass, your genetics, how much you move outside of formal exercise, your hormonal environment and dozens of other variables that no calculator can account for. Some people will find the estimate is close. Others will find it is out by several hundred calories in either direction. This is not a reason to avoid using one – a reasonable estimate is a far better starting point than guessing blind. Treat it as a starting estimate and refine it based on what actually happens to your weight and body composition.

If you have a fat-loss goal, then subtract 10–20 per cent from your TDEE for a sensible calorie deficit. This is enough to make consistent progress without being so aggressive that your adherence, your ability to eat socially, your relationship with food, your energy or your recovery suffer.

But don't treat this guidance as gospel. Think of it as a hypothesis rather than a fact: here is roughly what my body needs, and now I will test it against reality. If you eat at a 10–20 per cent deficit from that estimate for four to six weeks and see no change, the most likely explanation is not that fat loss is impossible – it is that your true maintenance is lower than the calculator suggested and your deficit is smaller than you think.

When it comes to setting calorie deficits, there are two questions I get asked the most:

What happens if I drop my calories too low?

Most women I speak to are trying to stick to 1,200–1,400 calories a day. They've usually heard someone else is sticking to these calories or they've put stats into a generic calculator and clicked 'rapid fat loss' OR they've decided to try and stick to their BMR calories (their basal metabolic rate; see page 12 for a reminder). Regardless, for a lot of women this is an unsustainable (and unnecessary) deficit. It's often too low to stick to with any kind of flexibility, so they inevitably give up or have binging episodes which bring their calories up.

Very low calories are very hard to sustain. The likely outcome is the restrict–overeat cycle: you are extremely rigid, you last a few days, you crack, you significantly overeat, you feel like you have failed, and you start again, but not before a few days of overeating and feeling sorry for yourself.

The heartbreaking thing is that you put in enormous effort to create a deficit and then overeat enough to cancel it out. You end up where you started but more exhausted and more convinced that something is wrong with you. Nothing is wrong with you. The deficit was just too aggressive and completely unsustainable.

Is calorie tracking accurate?

No. But this is not a reason not to do it. It does not need to be accurate to be effective. The most underrated benefit of tracking is simply awareness. People naturally eat less when they pay attention to what they are consuming, even before they make any deliberate changes.

One of the key behavioural shifts that happens when you start tracking is that you create a pause between seeing food and eating it. That pause is where the decision actually lives. It is worth far more than the calorie count itself.

If you've never calorie counted before

If this is new territory for you, here's how to start. Download a tracking app – at the time of writing, MyFitnessPal and Cronometer are both widely used and have large food databases. They're free to use at a basic level and that's all you need.

Search for the foods you eat and log them as you go. Most packaged foods can be scanned directly with your phone camera, which makes it faster than it sounds. For home-cooked meals, log the ingredients individually.

Use a set of digital kitchen scales to weigh your food, at least to begin with. Portion sizes are notoriously difficult to estimate accurately, and most people significantly underestimate how much they're eating – not out of dishonesty, just because eyeballing is really hard. Weighing for a few weeks builds a much more accurate mental map of what portions actually look like, and most people find they need to do it less rigorously once that foundation is in place.

Remember, you don't need to be perfect. You need to be consistent, accountable and honest with yourself. A friend once pointed out that your body is the most accurate food diary you ever keep. You can't cheat it.

Why Range Targets Beat Conventional Calorie Targets

One of the most common reasons people don't achieve their fat-loss goals is because they give up the moment they can't be perfect. You know the feeling: you've set yourself a strict daily target of 1,600 calories. You're doing well until Wednesday afternoon when a colleague brings in doughnuts or you grab something at the petrol station. Suddenly, you're at 1,650 calories. In your head, the day is 'ruined'. And because it's ruined, you might as well really ruin it. You eat the biscuits. You order the pizza. You decide to 'start again on Monday'.

This is an all-or-nothing mentality, and it is one of the biggest reason people don't get results. If you give up every time you miss your target, you will never get consistent results. Because life is never perfect. But the good news is you don't need to be perfect.

Think about it like playing darts. In the all-or-nothing mindset, you only get points if you hit the bullseye. Miss by a millimetre? Zero. That's an almost impossibly demoralising way to play a game – and yet it's exactly how most people approach fat loss.

In reality, darts doesn't work like that. You still score if you hit the 20. You still score in the treble. You're still in the game. You're still moving your score forward. You might not get the maximum at every turn, but you never score zero just because you didn't hit the exact centre.

Whenever I set calorie targets for clients, I don't give them a single static number. That sets people up to fail. Instead, I give them a range with two ends – what I call 'range targets'. When there's no single number to fail against, you stay consistent. And consistency, not perfection, is what produces lasting results.

How Range Targets Work

At one end is the Optimal Target, which is what you're aiming for on your good days – when you've slept well, your stress is manageable and you have the time and energy to give it your best. This is where you make your fastest progress. This target should be hard enough to push you and challenge you.

At the other end is the Non-Negotiable – this is your minimum effective dose. It is the target you hit on your hardest days – when you're exhausted, emotional, stressed or just generally can't be bothered. I think of this as a personal standard: 'I will at least do this, no matter what.' By always hitting your Non-Negotiable, you're always moving forward, just sometimes more slowly. Sticking to this is a form of self-respect and becomes part of your identity: 'I show up for myself.'

Let's look at how this works with calories. Let's say your maintenance is about 2,000 calories. To lose fat, your Optimal Target would be 1,600 – a solid deficit that produces good progress. But some days, 1,600 might feel impossible, or maybe you have a nice brunch and dinner planned and it's going to push you over that. So, you set a Non-Negotiable maximum of 2,000. Here's the key insight: anything under 2,000 is still a deficit. If you eat 1,800 calories, you haven't 'ruined' anything. You're in a smaller deficit. But it is still a deficit and you're still losing fat. You're still on track. You're still moving forward. The question is just how fast – not whether you're progressing.

You can also use the same principle when it comes to setting targets for your workouts or step count. For example, say your Optimal Target is 12,000 and your Non-Negotiable is 8,000. On a difficult day, you focus on hitting 8,000 – not on the 4,000 you're 'missing'. You take a short walk at lunch, pace during a phone call and park further away. You hit your minimum and go to bed having moved forward, not backwards.

There is a reason I have picked these numbers as examples. The vast majority of health benefits come from the first 7,000–8,000 steps you do per day. After that, the benefit tends to plateau. It's not that there is no more benefit, but the benefit becomes smaller and smaller per extra effort input. An Optimal Target for fat loss of 12,000 steps is a good target as expenditure is high but not so high that it starts to ramp up hunger and make it harder to stick to a deficit.

It's important to note here that 12,000 steps as an Optimal Target is an aspirational target, not a daily minimum. If you are currently averaging 4,000 steps, trying to jump to 12,000 overnight is often unrealistic. A better approach is to add 1,000–3,000 steps to your current average and build from there over several weeks. In same breath I want to tell you not to underestimate yourself. Many of my clients go from doing 6,000 to 12,000 steps a day and didn't believe they could until they decided to try. When setting your own range targets, make sure you're not creating ceilings for yourself.

The Science Behind It

Setting range targets is built on the research around flexible dietary restraint versus rigid restraint. Studies consistently show that people who adopt a flexible approach to their eating and exercise habits are significantly more successful at long-term weight management than those who are rigid.

Rigid restraint – the all-or-nothing approach – is associated with higher levels of stress, disordered eating and a greater likelihood of abandoning the whole approach after a minor setback. Adaptive goals, which adjust based on your current capacity and circumstances, have been shown to outperform static goals for long-term behaviour change. When your goal feels achievable given where you actually are today, you're more likely to take action. When it feels impossible, you're more likely to give up before you start.

The beauty of this system is that it removes the guilt of not being perfect. If you're having a bad day and you're struggling to function, aiming for 10,000 steps might feel genuinely impossible. And when a goal feels impossible, the likely outcome is doing nothing at all. But if you know that your Non-Negotiable is, say, 4,000 steps, that feels achievable. You hit it. You go to bed having met your target. You feel like a success rather than a failure.

This builds what psychologists call 'self-efficacy' – your belief in your ability to do what's required. Every time you hit your target, you're reinforcing the habit of showing up. You're proving to yourself that you can be consistent even when things are hard. That evidence accumulates. And the accumulated evidence changes your belief about what you're capable of.

Remember: fat loss isn't won on your best days. It's won on your worst ones. It's won by not quitting when things get hard.

The Most Common Mistakes

The part people get wrong when they set their own range targets is setting an unrealistic Non-Negotiable. They make their 'minimum' so high that it's actually an Optimal Target in disguise. Then when they inevitably miss it on a difficult day, they fall right back into the all-or-nothing trap.

Remember these are your personal standards. These are the daily actions you have set for yourself and promised yourself you can do. If you set these too high, you end up breaking promises to yourself and that is a slippery slope. Your Non-Negotiable should be something you can hit on your absolute worst day. Not your worst day when you planned everything perfectly and got seven hours of sleep. Your actual worst day – a sick child, no sleep, back-to-back meetings and you didn't get home from work until 8pm. If you can't hit it on that day, it's not a Non-Negotiable. It's just a slightly lower Optimal. And on those days, give yourself some damn credit because that is hard. Those days where you hit your Non-Negotiable despite everything, they are the hardest days, they are when most people give up and they are far more impressive than the days you hit your Optimal Target and everything feels easy.

Once you've set a genuine Non-Negotiable, you have to be strict with it. I treat mine as a promise to myself. Non-Negotiable means non-negotiable – not 'unless I'm tired' or 'unless it's hard today'. There are obviously a few legitimate exceptions, like being unwell or needing to be there for a loved one, but you will know if it's an excuse or a genuine reason. Everything else: it's getting done.

Another mistake many people make is to subtract the 10–20

per cent from their BMR – aka their maintenance needs – rather than their TDEE. If you do this, you will be miserable and will find it totally unsustainable. For example, my BMR is about 1,300 calories. Therefore, if I subtracted 20 per cent from that, I would be trying to eat close to 1,000 calories a day – no thank you. But my estimated TDEE is 2,100 calories so a sensible deficit is about 1,680 calories, which is much more sustainable!

Direction is more important than speed. Avoid trying to make your good days perfect and focus on making your bad days mediocre. You'll get better results this way.

KEY POINTS

- A deficit of 10–20 per cent of your total daily energy expenditure is a sensible, sustainable starting point for most people.
- Calorie tracking does not need to be accurate to be useful. The awareness it creates is most of the benefit.
- Flexible restraint consistently outperforms rigid restraint in long-term fat-loss research.
- The all-or-nothing mentality is the most common reason people don't get results – not genetics, willpower or lack of information.
- Range targets have two points: your Optimal Target (best days) and your Non-Negotiable (worst-case days). Both produce forward progress, just at different speeds. The idea is you have no days going backwards. The momentum is always forwards. This is how you get the fastest results.

- For fat-loss goals, remember: anything below maintenance is a deficit. Going to your Non-Negotiable on a hard day is not failure – you are still moving forward. Take the win.
- Every time you hit your target, you build self-efficacy. That accumulated evidence changes your belief about your own capability.
- Your Non-Negotiable must be genuinely achievable on your hardest days. If it isn't, it's not a Non-Negotiable. It's unrealistic and you start losing self-trust as you break the promise you have set to yourself.

PART 2

THE BULLSH*T FILES

Now that you understand how fat loss works, you are ready to see exactly what the industry has built on top of it. Part 2 is a rigorous, evidence-based dismantling of the most common myths, misconceptions and deliberate misinformation in the fat-loss world.

The goal of this part is not to make you angry, although you may be – I am sometimes! It is to give you a reliable filter that you can apply to any claim, any product and any influencer, for the rest of your life. By the time you finish Part 2, you will be able to spot misinformation within seconds – and you will understand why it was so convincing in the first place. My aim for this section is to make sure you never get scammed again.

Chapter 6

The Fat-Loss Myths

I spoke to a woman recently who had stopped going to her spin classes. She loved spin. It was the one part of her week that was just for her. She had been going for three years. And then she listened to a podcast, hosted by a doctor with a large following, who told her that spin raises cortisol too much for perimenopausal women and is negatively impacting their health. So she stopped. This is a tragedy.

Diet and exercise are the only universally agreed-upon interventions to improve menopause symptoms. The cardiovascular and metabolic benefits of exercise become *more* important as we age, not less. By quitting spin because of a claim that had no meaningful evidence behind it, this lady was removing something genuinely good from her life to protect herself from a risk that did not exist.

This is what misinformation costs women. Not just money, though it costs that too in money wasted on fad diets and supplements. It costs them years of healthy habits, disrupted by someone with a platform who sounded convincing.

I have spent years debunking poor health, fitness and wellness information on social media and, honestly, the noise has never been louder. Probably because the financial gain for these people has never been bigger. Confused people end up doing nothing or, worse, they do things that actively harm their health. So, in this chapter, I want to give you a framework for evaluating any fat-loss claim you encounter. By the end, you will be able to assess whether something is worth your attention, whether something is science or whether it is bullsh*t. But, first, let's get one thing clear . . .

Calling Out Misinformation Is Not Anti-Feminist

This is a hill I will die on. (Or possibly be killed on, judging by some comment sections on my social media pages.) More than a few times, I have been called anti-feminist for highlighting misinformation shared by women. But calling out false claims is not anti-feminist, even if the person making those claims is a woman. It is pro-truth. Pro-women. Pro-informed decisions.

If we are serious about empowering women, then we cannot selectively apply standards of evidence based on who is delivering the message, how nicely it is packaged or whether we think they seem like a nice person. Feminism, at its core, is about equality, autonomy and empowerment. Autonomy requires accurate information. You cannot make an informed decision if the information you are given is exaggerated, selectively presented, emotionally manipulated or simply lacks supporting evidence.

When women are sold supplements or protocols based on misinformation, fear or pseudoscience, their autonomy is being undermined. They are not making fully informed choices. They are reacting to amplified anxiety. That is not empowerment. It is persuasion and clever marketing dressed up as empowerment in order to exploit women.

How Misinformation Gets Wrapped in Empowerment

One of the uncomfortable realities of working in the female fat-loss space is that misinformation often comes wrapped in language that feels supportive. It speaks about finally understanding women's bodies. It criticises mainstream advice as being designed for men. It promises to validate the frustration so many women feel. And then, almost inevitably, it offers a product, protocol or specialist plan.

And most of these rely far more on clever marketing than on strong scientific evidence. The messaging is rarely neutral. It is urgent, emotive and often fear-based. The implication is that something inside you is malfunctioning and that you need to act quickly to correct it.

Calling this misinformation out protects women. It prevents them from wasting money on products or plans that promise physiological miracles but deliver minimal measurable benefit. It prevents them from blaming themselves when the promised transformation does not materialise. Because when the product fails, the narrative rarely shifts to the evidence being weak. Instead, the woman assumes she did something wrong, or that her body is uniquely broken.

Critiquing claims is not about gender. If a man made the same exaggerated claims, challenging him would not be anti-male. It would be pro-evidence. The same standard must apply here. Equality means holding everyone to the same evidentiary threshold. Lowering that threshold because the message is delivered by or aimed at women is not supportive. It is patronising.

There is also an important distinction between supporting women and blindly supporting everything women do. True support respects women enough to expect honesty, integrity and accountability. It does not shield misinformation from scrutiny simply because it is delivered in the language of empowerment. Protecting women from exploitation is feminist. Normalising exploitation because the person profiting is a woman is not.

Why This Marketing Works So Well

It is also worth acknowledging why this marketing is so effective, because these are not stupid women being fooled. These are intelligent people responding rationally to an environment designed to make them feel inadequate.

Women are repeatedly told that their bodies are complicated, fragile and in constant need of management. From puberty through to pregnancy, postpartum and menopause, the messaging is consistent: your body is hormonal, unpredictable and requires specialised intervention.

This creates vulnerability. When you have been conditioned to believe that your physiology is unstable, a product promising control and simplicity is genuinely appealing. The marketing works not because women are gullible, but because it speaks directly to a very real, very exhausting experience of feeling like your body does not behave in the way it should.

Understanding this is part of the solution. The more clearly you can see the mechanism and understand the way it works, the harder it is to fall for it.

How to Spot the Bullsh*t

Whenever I hear a wild new claim, I ask these three questions, in order:

1. What specifically does this product claim to do? 'Supports health' isn't enough. What exactly is it claiming will change in your body?
2. Is there peer-reviewed evidence in humans, at the dose included in this product, that it does that thing? Not a testimonial. Not a compelling story. Not a before-and-after photo. Actual research, ideally not funded by the company selling the product.
3. Even if it does that thing, does that thing actually affect the outcome you care about?

That last question is the one most people skip. A supplement might genuinely increase collagen synthesis, but does increased collagen synthesis reduce body fat? It doesn't. However, if the marketing loosely connects those two things, and you want to believe it, it's easy to miss the gap. I will often ask women why they are taking a supplement and the most common answer I get is, 'I don't know.'

Most products fail at question two. The ones that pass question two often fail at question three. Very few survive all three.

The Bullsh*t Radar You Are Now Building

The goal of this chapter is not to make you cynical about everything you read. It is to give you a reliable filter.

Good information is usually unsurprising and sometimes quite boring. It does not promise fast results. It does not require expensive interventions. It tends to reduce complexity rather than add to it. It refers to logic you can understand and verify. It is comfortable saying 'we do not know yet' when the evidence is not clear.

Misinformation is usually exciting. It is urgent. It has a villain, often mainstream medicine or the diet industry, and a hero, usually the person selling you something. It promises to explain why everything you have been doing is wrong and how their approach is different. If it sounds too good to be true, it usually is. No, the random influencer you follow probably hasn't just found the secret to fat loss we have all been looking for.

We are now going to spend the next several chapters applying this filter to the most common myths in fat loss. Some of what follows will be familiar. Some of it will surprise you. All of it is grounded in the same principle: the truth is simple, the evidence is what matters and your intelligence deserves to be respected.

Confused people do nothing. Informed people take action.

KEY POINTS

- Calling out misinformation targeted at women is feminist, not anti-feminist. You cannot make an informed choice when the information you have been given is exaggerated, emotionally manipulated or unsupported by evidence. The same standard of evidence must apply regardless of who delivers a claim or who it is aimed at.
- Misinformation in this space almost always arrives wrapped in the language of empowerment. Recognising this makes you much harder to exploit.
- Apply three questions to every fat-loss claim. What specifically does it claim to do? Is there evidence, in people like me, at the relevant dose, that it does that thing? And even if it does that thing, does that thing actually affect fat loss?
- Misinformation is usually exciting and promises to explain why everything you have been doing is wrong. Good information, on the other hand, is usually unsurprising and sometimes quite boring.
- Confused people do nothing. Informed people take action. The point of building your bullsh*t radar is not cynicism – it is the freedom to act with confidence on what actually works.
- Be more sceptical when claims seem unlikely.

Chapter 7

The Starvation Mode Myth

You have probably come across the terrifying idea that if you drop your calories too low, or diet for too long, you will break your metabolism. Your body will enter 'starvation mode'; it will refuse to let go of fat because it does not feel safe and you will eventually reach a point where you cannot lose weight even on 800 calories a day.

It sounds scary. It sounds plausible. It often fits with how people feel, like they are sticking to low calories and not seeing the results they expected. And conveniently, the person telling you about it usually has a 'metabolic reset protocol' or a 'reverse dieting plan' to sell you for several hundred pounds.

I want to take the fear out of this and give you the truth. Your metabolism is not that fragile. It is a highly sophisticated, incredibly resilient survival machine. It does not break. It adapts.

Why Starvation Mode Cannot Work the Way They Describe It

Let me use some logic here. If starvation mode actually worked the way it is described on social media, where your body simply stops burning fat because your calories are low, no one would ever actually starve to death. People would just stop losing weight. That is clearly not what happens.

A famous, though extreme, example is Angus Barbieri. In the 1960s, under strict medical supervision at the University of Dundee, Angus did not eat a single morsel of food for 382 days. He lived on water, tea, coffee, vitamins and electrolytes. He started at 456 pounds and ended at 180 pounds. His body did not hold on to fat because it did not feel safe. It did exactly what bodies are designed to do when there is no food available: it used stored fat for fuel.

I am absolutely not suggesting you stop eating for a year. But Angus's story, documented in the *Postgraduate Medical Journal* in 1973, proves a fundamental principle: if you are in a genuine energy deficit, your body will use stored fat. It cannot do otherwise. This comes down to the laws of thermodynamics – specifically the first law, which states that energy cannot be created or destroyed, only converted from one form to another. In the context of your body, this means the energy you consume has to go somewhere, and the energy your body uses has to come from somewhere. If you are taking in less energy than you are burning, the shortfall must be made up from your stored energy – which, as you now know, is primarily body fat. There are no exceptions to this. It is not a dietary opinion or a coaching philosophy. It is physics. The laws of thermodynamics do not have an exception for women who are stressed about dieting. Your body cannot hold on to calories that are not there.

What Is Actually Happening: Metabolic Adaptation

The scientific term for what people are experiencing when they think their metabolism has broken is 'metabolic adaptation', sometimes called 'adaptive thermogenesis'. When you lose weight, your energy expenditure drops for three very logical reasons:

1. There is less of you. A smaller body requires less energy to move and maintain. Think of it like a car: a Mini uses less fuel than a Range Rover. When you lose 10kg, you are a smaller vehicle. You need fewer calories to maintain your now lighter body mass.
2. Your body becomes more efficient. It learns to do the same tasks while spending less energy. This is partly a function of fitness, one aspect of which is doing more with the energy available, and partly a consequence of being lighter and thus requiring less energy to move generally. Imagine carrying the 10kg of body fat you lost up the stairs with you – it's going to expend more energy, right?
3. Your NEAT (non-exercise daily movement) reduces. This is the big one. All the unconscious movement that makes up your day tends to drop when you are in a calorie deficit. Your body tries to conserve energy by subtly and unconsciously reducing how much you fidget, pace, gesture and move around. You usually do not notice this happening, but it can account for a meaningful reduction in your daily energy expenditure.

None of this is metabolic damage. It is adaptation. It is predictable, it is reversible and it does not mean your metabolism is broken.

So Why Does Fat Loss Slow Down?

If you have been in a deficit for a while and your progress has stalled, there are a few likely explanations. Your calorie needs have reduced as you have lost weight, so the deficit you were in is now smaller than it was. Your NEAT has dropped unconsciously, reducing your energy expenditure. And your tracking accuracy may have drifted over time: portions that were once weighed are now estimated, minor inaccuracies accumulate and your deficit becomes smaller.

You also lose less total weight when you have less weight left to lose. When you start a fat-loss diet, you tend to lose weight quicker. It makes sense as you have more to lose. Once you've lost a fair amount of weight, the rate of weight loss slows. You've done nothing wrong; nothing needs to change. This should be expected.

None of these situations require a metabolic reset. They require an honest reassessment of your current intake and expenditure, and sometimes modest adjustments to maintain your deficit.

I would only consider reducing calories for a client if weight loss has genuinely plateaued for two to three weeks, despite consistent adherence. This is not common. Many of my clients lose fat from start to finish without ever needing to reduce their calories, because the initial deficit was sustainable enough to stick to throughout.

The Real Cost of This Myth

Beyond being factually wrong, the starvation mode myth is genuinely harmful. It makes women afraid to diet, afraid to create a deficit and afraid to lose weight too fast. And it sells them expensive protocols to fix a problem that does not exist.

It also, perversely, encourages very low-calorie approaches by suggesting that any deficit will eventually stop working, so you might as well go hard. This is exactly the opposite of the truth. Moderate, sustainable deficits – like the range targets we discussed in Chapter 5 – work better over time than aggressive, unsustainable ones.

Your metabolism is not broken. It is doing its job.

Metabolic adaptation is real. Metabolic damage is not. Your body is adapting, not breaking. Those are very different things. Some metabolic adaptation is a normal and inevitable part of successful fat loss.

KEY POINTS

- Starvation mode, in the sense of your body refusing to lose fat despite a genuine calorie deficit, does not exist. It is a myth used to sell metabolic reset programmes.
- Metabolic adaptation is real: as you lose weight, your body becomes smaller and more efficient and uses less energy. This is normal and expected, not a sign of damage.
- NEAT tends to drop unconsciously during a deficit, reducing energy expenditure in ways you will not notice. This is one of the main reasons fat loss slows over time.

- If your progress has stalled, the most likely explanations are a reduced calorie need as you have lost weight, reduced NEAT or a drift in tracking accuracy, not a broken metabolism.
- Moderate, sustainable deficits consistently outperform aggressive, unsustainable ones. Your metabolism works better when you are not fighting it.

Chapter 8
The Cortisol Con

If you are a woman over 30 and spend any time on social media, you will have seen the cortisol posts. Usually, it is someone pointing to their midsection, explaining that the reason you cannot lose weight, specifically that stubborn belly fat, is because your cortisol is too high. They talk about adrenal fatigue, starvation mode (yes, it crops up here too) and the need to balance your hormones with an expensive supplement or a restrictive protocol. It sounds empathetic. It sounds like they finally understand why you have been struggling despite doing everything right. But it is scientifically misleading. And worse than that, it is deeply disempowering. I am here to give you your autonomy back.

What Cortisol Actually Is

Cortisol is not a bad hormone. It is absolutely essential for your survival. You would not want to reduce it to zero even if you could.

Cortisol is your body's primary stress hormone, but it does far more than just respond to tight deadlines and difficult conversations. It helps you wake up in the morning, which is called the cortisol awakening response. It also helps you focus, move and perform, and it keeps your metabolism running. Without it, you could not function.

Cortisol is part of a highly sophisticated feedback loop called the HPA axis, the hypothalamic-pituitary-adrenal axis. Your brain constantly monitors what is happening in your body and your environment and decides exactly how much cortisol is needed at any moment. If levels rise too high, your brain signals your adrenal glands to produce less. If levels fall too low, it signals them to produce more. Your body is very good at managing this on its own and has evolved over millions of years to do this. You do not need a supplement to do what your brain and adrenal glands are already doing perfectly well.

Does Cortisol Stop Fat Loss?

The idea that high cortisol puts your body into protection mode or starvation mode and physically prevents fat loss is another myth. A well-marketed, widely believed myth, but a myth all the same.

While it is true that chronically high cortisol can cause water retention, which absolutely can mask fat loss on the scales and can make you feel puffy, cortisol itself does not stop fat loss. If you are in a calorie deficit, you will lose body fat. Full stop.

Here is the thing that should settle this once and for all: some studies show that the stress of dieting itself increases cortisol levels. In those same studies, the participants still lost weight. If cortisol stopped fat loss, no one would ever successfully complete a diet, because the very act of dieting is a physiological stressor.

Stress Affects Your Behaviour and Your Behaviour Affects Fat Loss

There is an important distinction to make here, because stress *does* affect fat loss, just not through cortisol directly blocking it. Instead, chronic stress affects your behaviour. It disrupts your sleep, which increases hunger hormones. It reduces your motivation to train. It makes you more likely to reach for highly palatable, energy-dense foods like chocolate, crisps and ice cream as a coping mechanism. It reduces your cognitive bandwidth, making consistent decision-making harder. Those behavioural changes affect your energy balance. And, as you know, your energy balance determines your fat loss.

This is why the cortisol narrative is so disempowering. It makes you think the issue is a hormonal malfunction you have no control over, rather than a lifestyle that is consistently over-challenging your capacity to recover and a diet and exercise plan that is not suitable to your current lifestyle. If you are in a calorie deficit and not losing weight, the issue is not cortisol. The issue is almost certainly one of the following: you are not in as large a deficit as you think and thus not seeing the results you expect; water retention is masking fat loss on the scales; or you haven't yet given it enough time – fat loss is rarely linear, and two to three weeks is not enough data to draw conclusions. It's very common and human to see behaviours slip because you're chronically stressed. This is not a failing on your part but it also doesn't mean you're storing fat despite being in a deficit.

What to Actually Do About Stress

When people talk about balancing their cortisol, what they are usually trying to do is manage their stress response. Which is genuinely worth doing. Just not with supplements. And certainly not with avoiding exercise, which seems crazy, but is genuinely suggested under the narrative that exercise increases stress and thus should be avoided if you have high cortisol. I hope it's needless to say that this is awful advice and research actually supports the opposite of this. Exercise helps you deal with subsequent stress.

Trying to lower your cortisol with supplements or a diet protocol without addressing what is causing the underlying stress is like trying to put out a fire by disabling the smoke alarm. You might stop the noise, but the house is still burning.

The things that genuinely help with chronic stress are boring, unsellable and require much more effort than simply taking a supplement: adequate sleep, regular exercise, managing your workload, reducing alcohol, being around people you like and spending time outside. These are free and have substantial evidence behind them. They also happen to be the same behaviours that support fat loss directly.

The other huge oversight is that most people are just assuming they have high cortisol based on feeling stressed. This may or may not be true. If you are genuinely concerned about chronically elevated cortisol levels, the right move is a blood test through your GP, not a supplement or to let TikTok diagnose you based on some really normal human traits. There are conditions, such as Cushing's syndrome, where medical intervention is necessary. If that is a concern, please speak to a doctor and do not self-diagnose from a social media post.

Cortisol does not block fat loss. Chronic stress affects the behaviours that determine whether you are in a deficit. That is a solvable problem, and no supplement is required.

KEY POINTS

- Cortisol is an essential hormone. It is not the enemy. You cannot and would not want to eliminate it.
- Cortisol does not physically block fat loss. People in calorie deficits with elevated cortisol still lose weight. The evidence is clear.
- Cortisol is part of the stress response, but it is not blocking fat loss directly. It is affecting the behaviours that create a deficit.
- Addressing stress means addressing the source of the stress: sleep, workload, movement, support. Not taking supplements.
- If you are genuinely concerned about your cortisol levels, speak to your GP and get a blood test.

Chapter 9

The Glucose Obsession

You may not know what a continuous glucose monitor, or CGM, is, but you have almost certainly seen one: that small, white, circular patch on the back of someone's arm. Originally developed for type 1 diabetics who can't produce insulin and need to track their blood sugar closely, these devices have been rebranded as the ultimate wellness accessory for people who eat carbs and feel vaguely anxious about it – usually because they've been told that glucose is inherently bad and should be avoided at all costs. Spoiler: it's not and it's totally normal and healthy for glucose to rise and fall throughout the day.

Welcome to the glucose obsession. And with it, the latest version of a very old myth: that carbohydrates are making you fat, not because of the calories they contain, but because of what they do to your hormones, specifically insulin.

Let me outline the theory, before explaining why it doesn't hold up.

The Carbohydrate-Insulin Model

The idea goes like this: you eat carbs, your blood sugar rises and your body releases insulin to clear that sugar from your bloodstream. Insulin is an 'anabolic' hormone, meaning it promotes storage, so it locks down your fat cells and prevents fat burning. Therefore, if you keep insulin low by avoiding carbs, you'll lose fat effortlessly regardless of how many calories you eat.

It sounds scientific. It sounds logical. But it's wrong and it completely disregards the energy balance equation I explained in Chapter 1 (see page 11).

Multiple tightly controlled metabolic ward studies, where researchers control every single calorie participants eat, have shown that when calories and protein are matched, there is no significant difference in fat loss between high-carb and low-carb diets. You may already know this from your own experience. If you've ever lost fat while eating bread, pasta or rice, congratulations: you have personally disproven the carbohydrate-insulin model.

Your body is far smarter than this theory gives it credit for. You can lose fat on a high-carb diet if you're in a deficit. You can gain fat on a zero-carb diet if you're eating more energy than you use. Insulin is a signal, not an override. You can spike insulin all you want, but if there are no excess calories, there is nothing to store. You cannot store energy that isn't there. That one sentence alone debunks half the myths you'll encounter in this space.

Sometimes I will use the following analogy to explain it: think of insulin like the baggage handlers at the airport. Their job is 'storage', much like insulin. And the glucose is the bags. What do you think will happen if there aren't any more bags to load? They can't be loaded, right? Even if more and more baggage handlers (insulin) come to load them. The same is true when there are no calories to store, i.e. you're in a calorie deficit. It doesn't matter if there is a tonne of the storage hormone around. You still can't store the calories if they aren't there.

The CGM problem

The biggest issue with the current glucose monitor trend is that it pathologises a completely normal, healthy response.

When a healthy person eats carbohydrates, their blood sugar rises. This isn't a dangerous spike. It's your body doing exactly what it's supposed to do. Your pancreas senses the rise, releases insulin, and your muscles, liver and fat cells take up the glucose for energy or safe storage. The whole thing happens efficiently, automatically and is over within a couple of hours.

You often hear wellness influencers suggest that these rises are inherently damaging and lead to inflammation, ageing and weight gain. But for a non-diabetic, these temporary rises are well within your body's ability to manage. In fact, the anxiety created by watching every glucose fluctuation on a monitor is likely doing more harm to your health than the pasta itself.

We are taking people with perfectly functioning internal regulation systems and teaching them to outsource their intuition to a sensor. This does not improve health. It creates food anxiety and a deeply distorted relationship with carbohydrates.

Personalised nutrition companies promise to tell you exactly which foods are 'good' or 'bad' for you based on your individual glucose and fat responses. The science is genuinely interesting, but the application is often flawed – here's why.

Acute glucose responses don't predict long-term health outcomes. A food that causes a higher glucose rise in the short term isn't necessarily worse for your health or your weight. You also rarely eat foods in isolation. Adding protein, fibre or fat to a carbohydrate meal significantly blunts the glucose response, so testing foods individually tells you very little about how you actually eat.

And here's the one that really gets me: fruit causes a bigger glucose response than many processed snacks. Does that mean a bag of crisps is healthier than a banana? Of course not. But that's the logical conclusion of optimising purely for glucose response.

Perhaps most perversely, many low-glucose strategies involve adding fat to food to blunt the spike: a teaspoon of peanut butter on every slice of apple; butter on your bread. This does reduce the glucose response, but it also adds hundreds of calories. You could end up gaining fat while successfully keeping your glucose low. Optimising for the wrong metric leads to the wrong outcomes.

What Causes Insulin Resistance

As I explained in Chapter 1, insulin resistance is what happens when your cells become less responsive to insulin's signal, so the pancreas has to produce more and more of it just to do the same job. Over time, if the cells still cannot keep up, blood glucose remains elevated. This is the mechanism behind type 2 diabetes, and it is also associated with higher blood pressure, elevated triglycerides and increased fat storage – the cluster of problems sometimes called metabolic syndrome.

So, if carbs aren't the culprit, what actually drives insulin resistance? The primary driver in the general population is ectopic fat – fat stored where it should not be: in the liver, around the organs and in the muscle tissue itself. When your fat cells become overfull and can no longer safely store excess energy, that energy spills into the bloodstream and other tissues, physically interfering with the insulin signalling process.

This is why losing even a small amount of body fat, around 5–10 per cent, can have such a dramatic impact on metabolic health. It is not about the carbs. It is about total energy balance and the health of your fat storage capacity.

What Actually Helps Your Blood Sugar

If you want to improve your metabolic health and manage your blood sugar well, you don't need a patch on your arm. You need the behaviours that allow your body to manage glucose efficiently.

Exercise is the most underrated tool here. When you contract your muscles, you activate glucose transporters that pull sugar from the blood directly into the muscle cells. You don't even need insulin for this process. This is why resistance training and walking after meals have such a powerful effect on blood glucose, and why muscle mass is so protective of metabolic health.

Losing body fat reduces the ectopic fat that's interfering with insulin signalling in the first place. Eating a diet high in fibre and protein naturally blunts glucose responses. Getting adequate sleep matters because poor sleep impairs insulin sensitivity significantly.

Put simply, the best thing you can do for glucose control is stay lean and active, avoid long periods of sedentary behaviour, build muscle which is the biggest site of glucose disposal and, if you want a bonus, go for a walk after big meals as this will clear glucose quicker.

None of this requires a monitor. None of it requires cutting carbs. It requires the same evidence-based fundamentals on which this whole book is built.

You don't need to fear your blood sugar. You need to manage your energy balance, move your body, build muscle and eat enough fibre and protein. The rest takes care of itself.

KEY POINTS

- The carbohydrate-insulin model, the idea that insulin from carbs prevents fat loss, is not supported by the evidence. Calories still determine fat loss.
- A glucose rise after eating carbs is normal and healthy. It's your body working exactly as it should.
- CGMs and glucose-optimising apps can create food anxiety and distorted eating without improving health outcomes for non-diabetics.
- Insulin resistance is primarily driven by ectopic fat accumulation, not carbohydrate intake.
- The best tools for blood sugar management are exercise (especially resistance training), fat loss, fibre, protein and sleep. Not glucose monitors.

Chapter 10

Don't Buy Another Supplement Until You've Read This

I want to tell you about Claire. Claire came to me spending just over £200 a month on supplements. Collagen powder in her morning coffee. A greens powder she didn't particularly enjoy but took anyway. Two different probiotics because she'd read conflicting things online and wasn't sure which was right. Ashwagandha for stress. A bloating supplement she'd found through an Instagram ad. Magnesium. Vitamin D. Omega-3.

She was meticulous about all of it. She set reminders. She ordered on subscription so she'd never run out. She had been convinced she would be missing out if she didn't take them.

When I asked what evidence she had that any of them were working, she paused. She felt good, she said. But she'd felt pretty good before she started. She'd gained weight over the same period. Her energy was still inconsistent. Her digestion still bothered her and she'd actually been experiencing worse bloating.

Claire is not unusual. She might be at the more extreme end of the spectrum, but she is almost every woman I speak to. Side note: she was actually really excited to be included in this book because she wants her story to stop other women wasting so much money on supplements.

In this chapter, we'll look at how the supplement industry is counting on your willingness to invest in hope, packaged beautifully, how to uncover the real science amid the claims, and the four supplements that are most likely to make a real difference for women.

A £60 Billion Industry Built on Your Confusion

The global supplement industry is worth over £60 billion. It is one of the fastest growing consumer markets in the world, fuelled by selling solutions to problems that are often exaggerated, misunderstood or entirely fabricated. Think cortisol blockers, hormone reset protocols, gut health drinks, magic collagen blends, salty water (electrolytes) – each one is built around a compelling story that contains just enough truth to sound plausible.

But what most people don't know is that it is an industry that is almost entirely unregulated in terms of efficacy. In the UK and US, supplement companies do not need to prove that their product works before they can sell it. They need to prove it's safe, which is a completely different bar. They can make vague structure-and-function claims – 'supports gut health', 'promotes energy', 'balances hormones' – without a single clinical trial showing that their specific product does any of those things at the dose they've included.

Think about that for a second. Every other health product you take – paracetamol, contraceptives, blood pressure medication – has to prove it works before it reaches you. Supplements don't. The marketing does all the heavy lifting. And it is extraordinarily good marketing.

I've spent 15 years watching this industry and the formula barely changes – and in the age of the influencer, it's got better and better and more and more convincing. But there is something else that is specific to the supplement industry that it's important for you to understand . . .

The Dose Problem

Even when a supplement contains an ingredient that has real evidence behind it, the dose matters enormously.

Many products include an ingredient at a fraction of the amount used in the studies that found any benefit. They can list it on the label. They can build their entire marketing campaign around it. But the amount they've included wouldn't produce a measurable physiological effect. This is completely legal. And because most consumers don't know what dose of any given active ingredient is required to produce a result, they have no way to evaluate whether what's in the bottle they're buying is meaningful.

A good example is ashwagandha. There's genuine evidence that ashwagandha can reduce self-reported stress and modestly lower cortisol, but the effective doses in those studies were 300–600mg of a standardised root extract. Many products on the market include far less, or use a form of the herb that hasn't been tested. Same label. Very different product.

The same applies to magnesium. Magnesium glycinate and magnesium malate are well-absorbed forms with decent evidence behind them. Magnesium oxide – the cheapest and most widely used form – is poorly absorbed and largely excreted. Your body can't use what it can't absorb. Yet the manufacturers will still make the same claims.

This is one reason I would highly recommend avoiding blended supplements. These are usually underdosed and overpriced. They can also add in a tonne of ingredients and claim it's going to cure everything for you.

Let me say this again: calling out supplement misinformation protects women. Not just financially, though the average supplement user in the UK spends over £400 a year. But psychologically. Because the story that your body is hormonally chaotic and in constant need of correction is one that keeps women spending, doubting themselves and distracted from the things that actually work.

Women shouldn't be made to feel like they are missing out because they can't spend hundreds of pounds a month on supplements, so I want to be clear: you are not.

The supplement industry doesn't need to prove their products work before they sell them. They only need to prove they're safe (which most are as they are underdosed and don't actually do anything). Marketing does the rest.

The Science Versus the Bullsh*t

Let's now go through the most common supplements one by one. I want this to be the section you screenshot, share with a friend and come back to the next time you're tempted by a convincing Instagram ad.

I'll be straightforward about where genuine evidence exists – because some supplements do have it – and equally straightforward about where the marketing has run miles ahead of the science, because that is usually the case.

Collagen

The claim: collagen is the protein that makes up your skin, joints and connective tissue. As you age, your body produces less of it. Taking a collagen supplement will top up your stores, improve your skin, reduce joint pain and support your gut.

The science: when you consume collagen – whether from a supplement, bone broth or chicken skin – your digestive system breaks it down into individual amino acids. The same amino acids you'd get from consuming any protein source. Your body then uses those amino acids however it decides is most useful. It doesn't direct them specifically to your skin or your joints just because you consumed collagen; it distributes them based on current need.

Does that mean collagen supplements are completely useless? Some studies – most funded by collagen manufacturers, which should be noted – have shown modest improvements in skin elasticity and joint discomfort in specific populations. The effect sizes are small. The study quality is low. And the same benefit could almost certainly be achieved by simply eating adequate protein from any source, which is considerably cheaper. The other point to note when you see any studies that show the benefits of collagen is that they are not well controlled. By this I mean the studies compared collagen to nothing or collagen to a placebo which is usually a carbohydrate drink. They don't compare collagen to whey, for example. This would be a fairer match as you would then see if the benefits were coming from protein or specifically from collagen. To date, we do not have any evidence to support collagen being superior to simply eating enough protein. However, when collagen and whey are compared directly for body composition outcomes, whey consistently outperforms collagen for stimulating muscle protein synthesis. This largely comes down to amino acid profile. Whey is a complete protein and is particularly rich in leucine, the key amino acid that acts as the primary trigger for muscle protein synthesis via the mTOR pathway. Collagen, in contrast, is low in leucine and lacks the amino acid tryptophan altogether, making it an incomplete protein. This is a sciencey way of saying that not all protein supplements are equal. Collagen is missing the specific triggers your muscles use to repair and grow. Whey isn't. If muscle, recovery or body composition is your goal, whey is the better investment.

A good example is a trial carried out in 2020, which compared collagen protein to whey protein following resistance exercise in older women. Despite providing equal total protein, whey stimulated significantly greater myofibrillar protein synthesis than collagen. This is the process by which your body builds the contractile fibres inside muscle cells – the actual machinery that makes muscles work and grow. It is the key measure of whether a protein source is genuinely contributing to muscle building, and it is what determines long-term muscle mass and strength. The difference between whey and collagen was attributed to whey's higher essential amino acid and leucine content.

This is why, from a muscle-building or body composition perspective, whey (or any complete, leucine-rich protein) is a superior choice. Collagen may contribute amino acids to the overall protein pool, but it is not an efficient driver of muscle protein synthesis and is therefore a lower-quality protein source if your goal is strength or lean mass.

A 2019 review in the *Journal of Drugs in Dermatology* found that collagen supplements showed promising results for skin ageing, but also acknowledged that most studies were industry-funded, short-term and had small sample sizes. The most comprehensive study to date – a 2026 umbrella review from Anglia Ruskin University, bringing together evidence from 16 systematic reviews, 113 randomised controlled trials and almost 8,000 participants – found a clearer picture: there were real if modest benefits for skin hydration and elasticity, and significant relief from osteoarthritis symptoms, but no meaningful improvements in sports performance or post-exercise recovery. The researchers themselves noted that marketing often runs ahead of the evidence. That is a long way from the miracle product collagen is often sold as.

A more recent concern worth noting is that in 2026, a well-known supplement company claimed collagen was essential for life, that children should take it and that it would improve everything from mental health to gut function. None of those claims have meaningful evidence behind them. This is exactly the kind of leap from grain of truth to sweeping conclusion that this chapter is about.

What I'd suggest instead: hit your total protein target from food such as eggs, meat, fish, legumes and dairy. Your body will use those amino acids for collagen synthesis where needed – alongside everything else it needs them for, like building muscle. We'll talk more about how to get adequate protein in Chapter 17.

Greens powders

The claim: one scoop, several servings of vegetables, job done. Convenient, complete, problem solved. But the science tells a different story.

The science: a greens powder is not the same as eating vegetables. To create a powder, whole vegetables are dehydrated and processed at high temperatures, and that process degrades many of the key nutrients that make vegetables worth eating in the first place. Phytonutrients (the plant compounds linked to reduced inflammation and disease protection), fibre (which feeds your gut bacteria and keeps you full) and bioavailable vitamins (meaning vitamins in a form your body can actually absorb and use) are all significantly reduced or lost entirely. You're paying a premium price for a nutritionally inferior version of something you could simply eat.

There's also a subtler psychological effect worth being aware of. People who take greens powders often feel they've 'done their vegetables' for the day – and research suggests they actually eat fewer whole vegetables as a result. The supplement ends up substituting for the behaviour rather than supporting it.

Transparency is another concern. A 2023 independent audit of popular greens products found that the majority did not disclose the actual quantities of individual ingredients – listing them instead as part of a 'proprietary blend'. This means you have no reliable way to know whether any given ingredient is present at a dose that would have any meaningful effect.

What I'd suggest instead: eat more vegetables. If that feels hard, start small: one extra portion a day. Add spinach to a smoothie. Have a side salad. Build the actual habit rather than buying a product that ticks the box without delivering the benefit.

An extra benefit here is that eating whole fruit and veg is much more satiating and cheaper than an often wildly overpriced greens drink. The most popular version at the time of writing will set you back £79 a month.

Probiotics

The claim: take a daily probiotic and you'll support your gut health, boost your immunity, improve your mood, balance your digestive system and improve your fat loss all from one capsule.

The science: the gut microbiome is one of the most genuinely exciting areas of nutrition science right now. The research on how gut bacteria influence immunity, mood, metabolism and disease risk is fascinating and still developing. I want to be clear about that before I say what I'm about to say.

The leap from that genuine science to most probiotic supplements is enormous. Your gut contains trillions of bacteria from hundreds of different species in an ecosystem that scientists are still working hard to understand. Most probiotic supplements contain a handful of specific strains – often *Lactobacillus* or *Bifidobacterium* species – at a dose that may or may not survive your stomach acid and reach your large intestine in meaningful numbers.

A 2018 review in *Cell* found that standard probiotic supplements were actually outcompeted and cleared by participants' existing gut bacteria in many cases. The gut is not an empty house waiting for you to move in. It's already occupied, and it has strong views about new arrivals.

The evidence for specific probiotic strains in specific conditions – certain types of IBS, recovering from antibiotic treatment and some forms of infant colic, for example – is more promising. For general 'gut health' in a healthy person? Weak, very, very weak. Way too weak to be spending £79 for a four-week supply!

What I'd suggest instead: a diverse diet high in fibre, fermented foods (yoghurt, kefir, kimchi, sauerkraut) and reduced ultra-processed food. This has substantially more evidence for supporting a healthy microbiome than any probiotic supplement. It's also considerably cheaper.

Ashwagandha

The claim: take ashwagandha daily and you'll feel calmer, less stressed and more resilient – it's an ancient remedy with modern science to back it up.

The science: here's one that gets a different answer from me, because the evidence is actually more solid than most.

Ashwagandha is an adaptogenic herb used in Ayurvedic medicine, and several randomised controlled trials have found modest but real reductions in self-reported stress and anxiety. A 2019 study in *Medicine* found significant reductions in anxiety and cortisol in participants taking 240mg of standardised ashwagandha extract for 60 days compared to placebo. The effects were real.

My caveats: most of the research is in people with clinically significant stress, not the general population. The dose matters – 300–600mg of a root extract 'standardised to withanolide content' is what the effective studies used. Withanolides are the active compounds in the plant believed to be responsible for its stress-reducing effects – and standardisation means the manufacturer has tested and guaranteed a specific amount of them in every dose. Without that standardisation, the amount of active compound varies enormously depending on where the plant was grown, when it was harvested and how it was processed. A capsule that simply says 'ashwagandha powder 500mg' with no withanolide percentage on the label is a meaningfully different product from the ones used in the trials. You have no way of knowing whether you're getting an effective dose or very little of what actually worked in the research. Look for products that specify a withanolide percentage, or carry one of the branded standardised extract names: KSM-66, Sensoril or Shoden. Many products on the market don't specify this.

And the bigger point: if you have chronically high stress, a supplement that mildly reduces cortisol is addressing a symptom, not the cause. As we've seen, what actually reduces chronic stress is less glamorous: better sleep, reducing your workload, regular exercise and support from people around you. Ashwagandha can be a useful tool but it can't do the structural work.

If you want to try it, it's one of the few I wouldn't actively argue against. Just go in with realistic expectations and verify the dose. Please note that ashwagandha is contraindicated if you're pregnant or on thyroid medication.

Bloating and digestive supplements

The claim: take this supplement, drink this tea, follow this gut-reset protocol – and your bloating will disappear. This category is enormous, emotionally targeted and almost entirely unsupported by evidence for the vague claims being made.

The science: bloating is real and can be genuinely uncomfortable. But it's usually caused by specific, identifiable triggers: high-FODMAP foods – a group of fermentable carbohydrates found in things like onions, garlic, beans and certain fruits that some people's guts struggle to process – eating too quickly, swallowing air, or underlying conditions like IBS or coeliac disease. The solution to bloating is identifying your specific triggers, often through a structured elimination approach with a dietitian, not buying a supplement that claims to fix 'bloating' as a general concept.

Activated charcoal

This deserves a specific mention because it's everywhere right now, marketed as a daily detox and bloating remedy.

The claim: that taking it daily will 'detox' your gut, absorb toxins and leave you feeling lighter and less bloated.

The science: it *does* bind to substances in the gut – this is why it's used medically in poisoning cases, where you need to prevent the body from absorbing something harmful. But that same non-selective binding action means it binds to *everything* in its path: medications, nutrients, anything it encounters. Taking it routinely alongside food or other supplements is counterproductive at best. At worst, it reduces the absorption of medications you actually need.

What I'd suggest instead: if bloating is persistent and significantly affecting your quality of life, speak to your GP. It can be a symptom of conditions that deserve proper investigation, not a supplement.

Fat burners, metabolism boosters and weight-loss supplements

The claim: take a fat burner, metabolism booster or weight-loss supplement and your body will burn more fat, your metabolism will speed up and the weight will fall off faster. Some promise to suppress your appetite, block carbs from being absorbed or raise your body temperature to torch extra calories. The supplement industry wants you to believe that where diet and exercise have failed, there is a pill that will do the job.

The science: let me be brief here because the evidence is brief. There are no legal, over-the-counter supplements that produce meaningful fat loss beyond what a calorie deficit produces. None. Fat burners typically claim to work in one of three ways: increasing thermogenesis (raising body temperature to burn more calories), suppressing appetite or blocking nutrient absorption. Let's look at each.

Thermogenic ingredients – usually some combination of caffeine, green tea extract, capsaicin or synephrine – do raise metabolic rate slightly. Studies on green tea extract show an increase in energy expenditure of roughly 80–100 calories per day in some populations. Caffeine alone has a small, real thermogenic effect. But here's the problem: your body adapts. Within a few weeks, tolerance develops and the effect largely disappears. And caffeine is available in coffee which often has the additional benefit of suppressing appetite too.

Appetite suppressants vary wildly. Some fibrous products (glucomannan, for example) do have modest evidence for short-term appetite reduction. But 'modest evidence for short-term appetite reduction' is a long way from 'fat burner'. The effect sizes are small, the research quality is often poor and none of it substitutes for the dietary habits that actually create a sustainable deficit. You would be far better off following the guidelines in this book.

Carb blockers – typically white kidney bean extract – inhibit the enzyme that breaks down starch. In theory, this means some carbohydrates pass through undigested. In practice, the effect on actual calorie absorption is small and inconsistent, the gastrointestinal side effects (bloating, gas, diarrhoea) are common and the evidence for meaningful fat loss is not there.

Weight-loss medications are a completely different category. The 'GLP-1 receptor agonists' Ozempic, Wegovy and Mounjaro are a class of medication that mimics the hormone glucagon-like peptide-1 (GLP-1), which your gut releases naturally after eating to signal fullness to the brain and slow the rate at which your stomach empties. They work in a real and well-understood physiological way, have robust clinical trial data and require medical supervision. They're not supplements; they're prescription medications. The distinction matters. But yes, these work. They reduce appetite significantly by mimicking gut hormones that signal fullness to the brain. The result is a meaningful, sustained calorie deficit – not through willpower, but through genuine physiological change. That's a completely different category from anything sold over the counter.

What I'd suggest instead: save your money. If you're spending £50 a month on a fat burner, that's £50 a month that could buy more protein, more nutritious food or contribute to working with a professional who can actually help you build lasting habits.

The Four Supplements That Actually Earn Their Place

After everything you've read above, it's time for the supplements most likely to produce genuine benefit for most women. This is a short list for a reason, and the impact is still modest. In fact, the following supplements are mainly useful to avoid deficiency.

Vitamin D

If you live in the UK and you're not supplementing in vitamin D between October and March, you're almost certainly deficient. The sun in Britain simply isn't strong enough during those months to produce an adequate amount through skin exposure. Vitamin D deficiency is associated with fatigue, low mood, impaired immune function and reduced bone health. The NHS recommends 10 micrograms (400 IU) daily, though many researchers argue 1,000–2,000 IU is a more effective target in winter. It's cheap, it's evidence-based and there's no real debate.

Omega-3

If you're not regularly eating at least two portions of oily fish – think salmon, mackerel, sardines and herring – a week, an omega-3 supplement is worth considering. Omega-3 fatty acids (specifically EPA and DHA) have solid evidence for reducing inflammation, supporting cardiovascular health and improving triglyceride levels (as a reminder, triglycerides are the main type of fat that circulates in the blood, and high levels are a marker of increased cardiovascular risk). There's also reasonable evidence for mood and cognitive function. The evidence for fat loss directly is weak, but the general health case is strong. Aim for a combined EPA and DHA dose of at least 500mg per day, from a reputable fish oil or algae-based supplement if vegan or vegetarian.

Creatine

Creatine monohydrate is the most researched supplement in sports science – thousands of studies over decades – and the evidence is extremely solid for supporting strength, power output and muscle gain when combined with resistance training. For women specifically, research shows it can help maintain muscle mass during fat-loss phases, which matters – and we'll come on to why in Chapter 17. The cognitive benefits are more recent and still developing: some studies show improvements in memory and processing speed, particularly in sleep-deprived individuals, but this evidence is less settled than the strength data.

The standard dose of creatine monohydrate is 3–5g per day, and it doesn't need to be 'cycled' or 'loaded', which means you don't need a high-dose 'loading phase' to get started, and you don't need to stop taking it periodically. Just take 3–5g daily, consistently. Any product telling you otherwise is usually selling you a more expensive version of something that works perfectly well in its simplest form. If you're strength training, this is probably the most evidence-backed performance supplement there is.

As usual, the claims are often overstated. The effect is there but it is modest. Don't expect anything drastic. Just like you wouldn't from taking a vitamin. There are also many brands putting huge mark-ups on their 'specially formulated' creatine.

There is no need for this. Creatine monohydrate is well absorbed and the most studied source. Go for this and avoid being oversold.

Protein powder

Though this is not a supplement in the traditional sense, it is worth mentioning here: if you're consistently struggling to hit your protein target from whole foods alone – which, as I'll explain in Chapter 17, is genuinely difficult for many women – a protein powder is a pragmatic solution. Whey protein is the most studied and has the best leucine content for muscle protein synthesis. Plant-based blends (soy or pea and rice combined) are a reasonable alternative. Think of it as food in a convenient format rather than a tablet you're taking for a specific effect and use it to close the gap, not as a replacement for eating actual protein.

And that's the list. There may be others that you could benefit from in certain situations – for example, vitamin B12 if you are vegan or vegetarian and not getting it from your diet, or beetroot juice if you're an endurance athlete looking for an edge – but generally most people who have a varied diet do not need more. Any other supplements should be scrutinised hard before you spend money on them. Though I would also add that many women are low in iron – not anaemic, but low and this is worth getting checked with your GP.

There are four supplements with genuine evidence: vitamin D in winter, omega-3 if you're not eating oily fish, creatine if you're strength training and protein powder if you can't hit your target from food. Everything else needs to earn its place.

KEY POINTS

- The global supplement industry is worth over £60 billion and is not required to prove efficacy before selling products. Safety and effectiveness are two very different standards.
- Even when an ingredient has evidence behind it, the dose in the product often doesn't match the dose used in research. The label and the science can be very different things.
- The four supplements worth considering are: vitamin D in winter, omega-3 if you're not eating oily fish, creatine if you're strength training and protein powder if you're struggling to hit your protein targets from food.

PART 3

THE MINDSET SHIFT

We've reached the part that determines whether any of the knowledge you've accumulated so far – the science of fat loss and how to identify misinformation – actually translates into lasting change: your mindset. And before you glaze over, I'm not talking about manifesting, or positive thinking your way to a smaller waistline, or anything remotely fluffy. I'm talking about hard science. Part 3 is all about the evidence-based psychology of behaviour change, applied to fat loss.

The chapters that follow cover the things that will make or break your progress regardless of how good your plan is: your mood, the stories you tell yourself and the power of your own expectations. Each one has measurable physiological consequences that go far beyond what most people consider.

Knowing what to do is one thing; let's now get you in the right head space to take action.

Chapter 11

Mood First

I'm going to start this chapter by saying something that is often overlooked: if you want better fat loss results, a better body and a better life, you need to prioritise your mood.

Not motivation. Not discipline. Not willpower. Your mood. This is what determines your actions far more than any amount of grit or determination.

I spend my professional life talking to people who 'know what to do' but aren't doing it. If knowledge were the problem, this would be an easy fix. Most people know that fat loss requires eating less than you expend and moving your body more. If you've read Part 1, you know this too. But knowledge alone won't get you results. The reason fat loss feels so hard is not because people lack information, it's because fat loss is simple, but not easy. We confuse those two things constantly.

The real question isn't, 'What should I do?', it's, 'How do I make myself consistently do the things I already know will work?' Usually, people think the answer is a stricter plan, a new supplement or obsessing over their calorie target. But what largely determines whether you follow through, day after day, is your mood. Your mood shapes your decisions. Your decisions shape your habits. Your habits decide your results.

The good news is that mood is not something that simply happens to you. It is, to a meaningful degree, something you can influence. Not perfectly, not always and not completely, but more than most people realise. Sleep, sunlight, connection, gratitude – these are all fat-loss tools because they impact your mood, alongside the more obvious ones like movement, food and exercise. When you prioritise them, you are not just supporting your physiology. You are actively shaping the mental environment in which every food decision gets made.

Understanding that your mood drives your choices doesn't make you a passive observer of your own behaviour. It gives you a new lever. Instead of asking, 'Why can't I just stick to it?', you start asking, 'What's actually going on with my mood right now, and what can I do about it?' That is a far more useful question. And it has far more useful answers. I would also note here that your mood is not always a good representation of reality. You don't always need to act based on your mood and often (especially during PMS) it's better to ignore your mood and stick to what you know you need to do to get the result you're working towards.

In this chapter, we'll look at why mood is the hidden driver of every decision you make about food and exercise, and how to prioritise it deliberately.

Stop Treating Happiness as a Future Outcome

Think about the last time you were in a genuinely good mood. Things felt easier. Problems felt solvable. You had perspective. You were more patient, more resilient and it was easier to make choices that aligned with your goals.

When you're in a good mood, very little feels overwhelming. You're more likely to act, more likely to try again when something doesn't work and far less likely to catastrophise small setbacks. In contrast, when your mood is low, everything feels heavy. The smallest inconvenience feels impossible. You're more reactive, more impulsive and more likely to quit. This isn't just your experience – it's backed by science.

Shawn Achor's research, summarised in *The Happiness Advantage*, demonstrates something counterintuitive: happiness doesn't come after success. It comes before it. People who are happier are more productive, more creative, better at problem-solving and more resilient. They aren't happy because they've achieved more – they achieve more because they're happier. Positive affect literally expands the brain's ability to think, plan and persist.

Happier people look 'luckier' from the outside. In reality, they're just more willing to keep going – they're looking for solutions, staying open to opportunity and persisting through setbacks. The happiness comes first and the outcomes follow. This has direct implications for fat loss. If you approach the process from a place of frustration, self-criticism and deprivation, you're stacking the cognitive and emotional odds against yourself before you've taken a single action.

One of the most effective ways to shift this is to stop saying, 'I'll be happy when I've lost the weight.' That framing makes happiness conditional on an outcome you don't yet have. It also means you'll spend the entire process – whether that's months or years – putting up with some level of discomfort. And your ability to tolerate that discomfort will vary day to day, depending on your sleep, your stress levels and what else is happening in your life. Some weeks you'll feel completely fine. Others, the same calorie deficit will feel unbearable. That's normal – and knowing it's normal makes it easier to sit with.

No one feels good all the time, so you should never put off happiness for the sake of any goal – especially fat loss. When you do that, the goal becomes something to endure rather than something to pursue with any real enjoyment. So, stop treating happiness as a future outcome and start recognising what you already have. A simple daily practice of writing down two or three things that went well, or that you are grateful for, has been shown to meaningfully improve mood and reduce the negativity bias that keeps people stuck. It doesn't need to be elaborate. It just needs to be consistent. That is how you rewire your brain to be happier. This shift alone can change how the whole process feels.

There is also a belief worth breaking down here that many people consciously or subconsciously hold: the idea that your 'real life' starts when you hit your 'goal weight', or at least that life will be totally different. That you'll book the holiday then, wear the dress then, feel confident in your body then, start dating and find the perfect partner then. This is one of the most quietly damaging patterns I see, because it puts everything good on hold while you get there. Life is too short for that! And it doesn't work in the way you think it will.

Research on what's called the 'impact bias' consistently shows that people overestimate how much better they'll feel once a goal is achieved. The emotional high is real, but it's shorter and smaller than anticipated, and the background conditions of your life remain largely unchanged. The confidence you're waiting for doesn't arrive with the number on the scales. It arrives through the process of showing up for yourself, repeatedly, over time. Which means it's available to you now.

So don't wait. Book the holiday. Wear the dress. Go to the reunion. Ask them on the date. Live the life you're trying to lose weight for – while you lose the weight. Create the deficit, do the work and simultaneously refuse to defer your happiness to a future version of yourself that has it all figured out. That version of you is built from how you live today, not what you weigh at the end of it.

Mood and Food Are a Two-Way Street

Your mood affects what you eat and what you eat affects your mood. This feedback loop is one of the most powerful – and most underappreciated – drivers of success or failure when it comes to fat loss.

Research on how mood affects food choice reveals something important and counterintuitive: it is not just that you reach for the chocolate when you feel bad. It is that your emotional state changes the way your brain evaluates food at a structural level. A series of studies on mood and food preference found that people in a positive mood consistently made different food choices than people in a neutral or negative mood – specifically, they were more likely to choose options aligned with their longer-term goals rather than their immediate comfort.

The researchers link this to how mood affects what psychologists call 'temporal construal' – how far into the future your decision-making is oriented. A good mood appears to orient you towards longer-term thinking ('I want to feel healthy'), while a low mood pulls you towards the immediate ('I just need to feel better right now'). This is why the advice to 'just eat well and you'll feel better' is not wrong, but it is incomplete – it misses the direction of causation. Mood shapes food choice, not just the other way around. A woman who is chronically exhausted, over-stretched and running on high stress is choosing poorly because her brain is in a state that makes those choices predictable.

But a low mood doesn't just mean poorer food choices, it also leads to less movement (exercise requires activation energy that low mood depletes) and worse sleep (which then makes mood worse the next day). Those behaviours reinforce the low mood, and the spiral continues. Research from University College London found that higher consumption of ultra-processed food was associated with a significantly increased risk of depressive and anxiety symptoms, but, once again, the relationship also runs the other way. Low mood increases the desire for exactly those foods.

We often treat mood as something that just happens to us, like the weather – something we wait out and hope improves. But mood is something you can actively influence. It is, to a meaningful degree, a responsibility.

You Don't Wait for a Good Mood – You Create One

This is where imperfect action comes in. You don't wait to feel motivated and then start. You do the things that create a better mood and motivation follows. This sounds backwards until you experience it.

Behavioural activation – the idea that action precedes motivation, not the other way around – is one of the most replicated findings in behavioural psychology. Knowing this allows you to use it to your advantage. Here's how you can apply it in everyday life: keep a very short list of things that reliably shift your mood – a specific playlist, a podcast (the *ESGfitness* podcast is great, I hear), a ten-minute walk, a phone call with someone who energises you, a ten-minute workout or breathwork exercises. This is not meant to turn into a general self-care list. It's specific things that work for you in the immediate term. When your mood and/or motivation is low, go to the list and take some action. You'll be amazed at how a ten-minute workout can change your whole mood, energy and day.

Another practical framework I use to boost mood is to reframe the resistance – low motivation isn't a sign that something's wrong. It's a completely normal feature of doing hard things over a long time. Most people interpret resistance as a signal to stop. It's actually just friction – the ordinary cost of doing anything that matters. Recognising that the feeling of not wanting to do something is normal and expected makes it easier to deal with. I go one step further with this. If it's hard, it excites me more, because this is when most people give up. And most people never achieve their goals – because they give up way too soon. They give up on the days they don't feel like doing it. If you know that you will have those days from the start, if you accept that they are an inevitable part of achieving anything hard and that nothing worth having ever comes easy, then you embrace the hard work.

Finally, the ten-minute rule is the most reliable tool I have found for imperfect action, broadly supported in productivity and behavioural psychology. Tell yourself you'll do ten minutes of whatever you're resisting – the workout, the meal prep, the walk. Not 30 minutes. Not an hour. Just ten minutes. Almost always, once you've started, you'll continue. The activation energy required to begin is the hard part. Once moving, momentum takes over.

What starts as a decision to do a ten-minute walk can turn your whole day around.

Stop waiting to feel motivated and start focusing on your mood. If you can improve your mood by even 10 per cent, everything else – the training, the nutrition, the patience with slow progress – becomes measurably easier. Mood first. Everything else follows.

You have more control over your mood than you think.

KEY POINTS

- Mood determines behaviour far more than knowledge or discipline. Most people who 'know what to do' and aren't doing it have a mood problem, not an information problem.
- Happiness precedes success, not the other way around. Approaching fat loss from a place of frustration and deprivation makes every step harder. The more you can approach it from a place of genuine expectation rather than braced resignation – expecting to find it hard sometimes but also expecting to succeed – the more that expectation shapes what actually happens.

- Mood and food are a feedback loop. Low mood drives poor food choices; poor food choices worsen mood. The loop works in both directions.
- Don't wait for a good mood to act. Take the action that creates the good mood. The ten-minute rule is the most reliable tool for breaking inertia.
- A 10 per cent mood improvement changes the entire landscape of the day. Prioritise it deliberately, not as an afterthought.

Chapter 12

The Story You Tell Yourself

Sometimes – a lot of the time – it's not the calories, the workouts or the fad diets that are holding you back. It's the story you tell yourself.

We all have a narrator in our heads. A constant internal voice that interprets everything we do, everything we experience and everything we see. It tells you who you are, what you're capable of and – most damagingly – what you're not capable of. So much of how we experience life is defined by the story we choose to tell and where we choose to put our focus.

If you tell yourself the story that you've always failed, your brain will dutifully scan your memory for every piece of evidence that confirms it. It will replay the time you gave up on the keto diet, the gym membership you used twice and the weekend you 'ruined' with an entire packet of biscuits. If you're looking for evidence of failure, you will find a mountain of it with very little effort. Psychologists call this 'confirmation bias' – the tendency to seek out information that confirms what we already believe and to dismiss evidence that contradicts it. It's why the same set of results can look like failure to one person and progress to another.

But you could just as easily tell yourself the story of your successes: the times you showed up when you didn't want to; the times you chose the salad because it made you feel better; the times you handled a stressful week without turning to food. We rarely give ourselves credit for these moments – we feel we 'should' just do them, so they don't count. But they do. And the story you choose to tell yourself becomes a self-fulfilling prophecy.

The Physiology of Belief

In a study by psychologist Alia Crum and her team at Stanford, participants were given a set meal and had their ghrelin (a hormone that signals hunger to your brain) levels measured before and after. Then they were told (falsely) whether they had a 'high-risk' or 'low-risk' genetic profile for obesity and weight regain. The participants who were told they had the protective 'low-risk' variant showed a two and a half times greater rise in satiety hormones after the same meal than those told they were 'high-risk' – regardless of their actual genetic profile. Their bodies responded to the story they'd been told, not to their biology.

The researchers did the same thing with exercise. Participants were given fake information about their genetic predisposition for endurance, then retested on a treadmill. Those told they had 'bad' genes for exercise performed significantly worse the second time: their lung efficiency dropped, they fatigued sooner and they quit the test earlier. These are not things you can consciously control. You can't will your VO2 max (a measure of your cardiovascular fitness, specifically how much oxygen your body can use during intense exercise; the higher it is, the fitter you are) or your ghrelin levels to change. But your beliefs about your body can.

Other studies on athletic performance have found that cyclists who were given a placebo but told it was caffeine improved their time trial performance at the same level as those who actually received caffeine – the belief that something would help them perform better produced the same physiological benefit as the substance itself. Crum has also shown that people who hold the belief that stress is enhancing rather than harmful have a measurably different cortisol response to a stressor than people who believe stress is damaging. Not just a different experience of stress. A different biological response to it, measured in blood.

Taken together, this body of research makes one thing very clear: your thoughts about your limits are often more limiting than the limits themselves. If you expect to fail because of your 'bad genetics' or your 'slow metabolism', you are literally talking your body into performing worse.

The story you tell yourself about your body, your capacity and your history with food and exercise isn't just shaping your mindset, it is shaping your biology.

The Self-Fulfilling Loop

The story you tell yourself is dangerous because it directly influences the actions you take, which then reinforce the story. If you believe you won't be successful, why would you be fully motivated to put in the work required? You wouldn't. So you half-commit. You try a few things without full investment. You don't get the results. And then you tell yourself: 'See? I knew

I couldn't do it.' And the story grows more entrenched. More 'true'. More fixed.

One of the most common versions of this I hear – and one of the most damaging – is this: *I've tried this so many times and never got to where I want. What's the point in trying again?* But all this story is telling you is that every previous approach you tried was wrong for you. That's it. Whether it's true or false is irrelevant. And since the story is subjective anyway, you can choose to believe the narrative that is conducive to the outcome you want.

This is why it's often easier to coach younger people as they haven't spent decades reinforcing negative loops. When you've spent 30 years telling yourself you're 'not a gym person' or that you 'always fall apart at weekends', that story feels like a fundamental truth. Like your identity. But it's not. It's just a script you've been reading for a long time. And you can change it at any point.

Taking Ownership Without Blame

Realising you are the author of your own story is both empowering and daunting. Daunting because it means you can't fully blame your genetics, your upbringing or your 'slow metabolism' for where you are. Empowering because it means you have the power to change it.

Taking ownership doesn't mean taking the blame. You didn't choose your genetics. You didn't choose the environment you grew up in, the eating habits modelled for you or the years of restrictive dieting that may have warped your relationship with food. Those things happened and they matter. But you can choose to take ownership of your response to them. That's where your power lives – in the response, not the original cause.

If you've told yourself the story that you are 'just how you are' and can't change, then of course motivation feels absent. Motivation follows action, and action follows belief. You have to believe change is possible before you'll invest in pursuing it. Not blindly or naively – just enough to try. And trying, done with the right strategy, produces results. Results then change the story from the inside.

How to Start Rewriting Your Story

First: write down the story you're currently telling yourself about why you haven't been successful. Is it that you're lazy? That you love food too much? That you don't have the willpower? Get it out of your head and onto paper.

Then question it. Break it down the way you would for a friend. Are these stories objectively true? Are they helpful? Why do you think you've failed before? Usually, because previous attempts were too restrictive, too all-or-nothing, relied on motivation that was always going to run out or measured progress only by the numbers on the scales. You didn't fail because you're incapable. You failed because the plan set you up for failure.

Now get practical: prove yourself wrong. Outline what someone who isn't lazy would do. Maybe it's 8,000 steps a day, getting in a workout three times a week or making a healthy evening meal instead of ordering a takeaway. Then prove that you can do that.

Then take it further. Ask yourself, today: what would someone who has the results I want do in this situation? What would the fit, lean, healthy version of me do? And then do that. You don't think your way into a new story. You act your way into it, one decision at a time, until the evidence becomes impossible to argue with.

Most importantly, stop speaking to yourself as though your lack of success is a character flaw. It isn't. Every single person is capable of changing their body composition. It is not easy. But it is possible. And the people who get there aren't more disciplined than you and they're not built differently. They just stopped treating fat loss as something to endure and started living the way they needed to live long term – from the beginning. Sustainable calories. Realistic training. A plan that fits inside their actual life.

Be careful what stories you're telling yourself. None of them are objectively 'true' – they're interpretations. So you might as well choose the one that actually gets you where you want to go.

That's what makes this time different.

You didn't fail because you're incapable. You failed because the approach set you up to fail. That's a strategy problem, not a character flaw. There's a difference. You are limiting yourself more in imagination than in reality.

KEY POINTS

- The story you tell yourself produces measurable physiological effects – beliefs about your body change how it actually performs, including hunger hormone responses.
- Negative self-stories become self-fulfilling: they reduce effort, which reduces results, which reinforces the belief. The loop runs in both directions.
- Taking ownership of your situation is not the same as taking the blame for it. Ownership is where your power lives.
- Previous failure is almost always a strategy problem, not an ability problem. The plan was the issue, not you.
- You can choose your story. The empowering one and the limiting one are both available. Choose deliberately.

Chapter 13

The Expectation Effect

We've talked about how your mood shapes your decisions and why the story you tell yourself matters. There is one factor I haven't yet explained, and it's more powerful than those two things combined when it comes to determining your day-to-day experience of trying to lose fat.

That factor is the expectation effect, and it will blow your mind. Once you understand it, you can use it deliberately.

The Milkshake Study

Your hunger hormone ghrelin rises before a meal and drops after it. Most people assume this drop is determined by what you actually ate – the calories, the macronutrients, the physical volume. But that's not the whole story.

In a now-famous study by Alia Crum and colleagues at Stanford, participants were given the exact same milkshake on two separate occasions. The milkshakes were nutritionally identical – same calories, same fat, same protein. But the labels were different. On one visit, the shake was described as an indulgent, high-calorie treat. On the other, as a sensible, low-calorie diet drink. Ghrelin levels were measured before and after both.

When participants believed they were drinking the indulgent shake, ghrelin dropped sharply – a strong satiety signal. When they believed they were drinking the diet shake, ghrelin barely dropped at all. The food was identical. Only the expectation changed. Their bodies were responding not to what they ate, but to what they believed they'd eaten.

Crum and her team extended this with an omelette study. Participants were shown a recipe before eating – one group was told it contained four eggs, the other was told it contained two. The omelette actually contained three eggs for both groups. The group who believed they'd eaten the smaller omelette reported significantly more hunger two hours later and consumed substantially more calories over the rest of the day. The expectation shaped both their physiological hunger response and their actual eating behaviour that followed.

This is the perfect scientific explanation for why people find dieting so relentlessly hard. They approach it with a mindset of restriction and deprivation. Every meal is viewed through the lens of what they can't have. Every workout is punishment for what they ate. And their bodies respond accordingly: keeping hunger hormones elevated, keeping the 'this is not enough' signal running. It becomes a self-fulfilling experience.

The Hotel Cleaners

One of my favourite studies on the expectation effect comes from a completely different direction. Crum and fellow psychologist

Ellen Langer studied hotel room cleaners – women doing physically demanding work all day: making beds, scrubbing floors and lifting heavy linen. Objectively, they met the Surgeon General's recommendations for physical activity through their work alone. But when asked, most of them reported they didn't exercise enough. They didn't see their work as exercise. They saw it as work. That mental label changed everything.

Half were told simply: 'Your daily work meets and exceeds the recommendations for physical activity. You are getting a good workout.' The other half were told nothing. After just four weeks, the group whose mindset had been shifted – with no change in their behaviour, only their perception of it – showed significant physical improvements: weight loss, reduced body fat, lower blood pressure and improved waist-to-hip ratio. The control group showed nothing.

Now ask yourself, how often do you do the same thing? You walk somewhere but don't count it as exercise because it wasn't 'a proper workout'. You choose the salad but focus on what you're not having. You lift weights but tell yourself you're too old or too out of shape to make real progress. You are the hotel cleaner who doesn't believe her work counts – and your body is listening.

The Nocebo Effect

The expectation effect runs in both directions. The positive version – where positive expectations produce positive outcomes – is sometimes called the placebo effect. The negative version is the nocebo effect: where negative expectations produce negative physiological outcomes.

For example, take a high-pressure work week. You look at your diary on Sunday evening, see what's coming and tell yourself: *There's no way I'll be able to eat well or train this week.* That story is running in your mind before Monday has even started. As a result, you don't prep any food, because why bother. You skip the Monday workout because you know you won't have time to do a full hour. By Wednesday, you've been eating whatever's convenient, you haven't moved and your stress is high – partly because the things that help you manage stress (e.g. activity, exercise and good food choices) are the first things you dropped. You reach Friday and say: *See, I knew this week would be a write-off.*

Or take the new mum, running on broken sleep, trying to navigate a life that no longer resembles the one she planned for. The story is: *I can't prioritise myself right now. Everything is too chaotic. I'll get back to it when things settle down.* Except things don't 'settle down' and every week that passes adds another layer of evidence that this is just how life is now. She moves less, eats reactively, feels worse in her body, and the story gets louder: *I just don't have time for this.* The chaos of life is real. But the story that nothing is possible within it is not. You just need a different approach to when you had more time.

Or maybe you believe your metabolism has 'stopped working' because you're over 40. You will then unconsciously move less, eat less mindfully and behave in ways that confirm that belief. Your body responds by reducing energy expenditure. You then say: *See – I knew it was my metabolism.* And the prophecy fulfils itself.

Or perhaps you believe you have 'bad genes' for fat loss – Crum's research showed that people perform worse on endurance tests, show poorer physiological adaptation to training and experience less satisfaction from exercise all because of a fabricated genetic label. The gene doesn't determine the outcome. The belief about the gene does.

This is why the myths we've debunked throughout this book matter beyond just being factually wrong. The woman who believes her body is hormonally broken and beyond repair will invest less in it, expect less from it and get exactly what she expects.

Using the Expectation Effect Deliberately

Acknowledging the expectation effect isn't about lying to yourself. It's about choosing the most empowering and accurate interpretation of your situation. You can't think yourself lean, but you can choose the frame through which you experience the process:

- **How you label your food:** stop calling your meals 'diet food' or 'boring' or 'rabbit food'. Think of them as fuel – protein-rich, high-volume food that sustains your energy and keeps you full. The milkshake study tells you this label genuinely changes your hormonal satiety response.
- **How you label movement:** stop framing exercise as punishment. You are not 'working off' last night's dinner. You are building a stronger, more resilient body. You are investing in your future health and independence. You get to do this.
- **How you manage hunger:** understand what ghrelin actually is. When you feel hungry on a calorie deficit,

remind yourself that this is ghrelin doing its job. It is a signal, not a command. Tell yourself: 'I have fuelled adequately. This feeling will pass.' You don't always have to act on hunger. It is not a physiological emergency; it's a hormone that responds to context and expectation.

- **Give yourself credit:** actively focus on what you're doing right. Did you drink your water? Hit your protein? Go to bed on time? Choose the better option in a difficult situation? Every small win reinforces the belief that you are the kind of person who takes actions in line with their goals. Celebrate them. Write them down. Tell someone. Let yourself feel your wins. The brain responds to reward and recognition, and building a habit of noticing progress is one of the most underused tools in behaviour change.

Your body doesn't just respond to what you eat or how you train. It responds to what you believe about what you eat and how you train. That belief is something you can choose.

KEY POINTS

- Ghrelin – your primary hunger hormone – responds to what you believe you've eaten, not just the nutritional content of your meal. Expectation changes physiology.
- Hotel cleaners who were told their work counted as exercise showed measurable physical improvements within four weeks, with no change in behaviour – only mindset.

- The nocebo effect means that negative expectations produce negative physiological outcomes. Believing your body is broken or your metabolism is damaged can create exactly that reality.
- Label your food as fuel, not punishment or deprivation. Label movement as investment, not penance. These are not just mindset tricks – they change measurable outcomes.
- Give yourself credit actively and deliberately. Most people are wired to notice failures. Rewiring towards wins changes your belief about what you're capable of.

PART 4

YOUR FAT-LOSS TOOLKIT

Everything you've read so far has been building to this. You understand the science, you can cut through the marketing and you've spent Part 3 rewiring your mindset. Now it's time to connect everything you have learned into a way of living you can actually maintain. The tools I am about to explain are not a rigid 'programme' with a start and end date. They are principles that you will use for the rest of your life – adapted to wherever you are, whatever is happening and whatever your goals are at any given time.

Part 4 brings together the practical strategies that make fat loss feel manageable rather than exhausting. We'll cover everything from raising your energy, bad day management and habit automation to the importance of protein, sleep and hunger management. I'll also introduce you to a proven way to structure your eating day in a way that supports fat loss without having to track calories or obsess over food choices.

These tools are interconnected and designed to work together. By the end of this section, you will have everything you need to get in shape and live your life to the full.

Chapter 14

Start with Energy

I've spoken to thousands of women who know exactly what to do for fat loss but can't make it stick. When I ask why, the answer is almost always the same: 'I just don't have the energy.' You can have the perfect calorie target, ideal protein goal and best training plan, but none of it matters if you don't have the energy to execute it. We get fixated on tiny details – maybe our calories are 50 too high, maybe we need 5g more protein – when the real issue is that the foundation is not there. So, before we get into practical tools that will support you in your fat-loss journey, let's make sure you have the energy to do this. Most people don't consider this. Trying to change without first building your energy is like pushing a car with the hand-brake on, uphill (hard). Building your energy first is like rolling downhill with no brake.

Raising Your Energy Baseline

Trying to start something new from a place of exhaustion and stress is setting yourself up to fail. Yet time and again we do this to ourselves. And I'm not just talking about the 'I didn't sleep well last night' kind of low energy. It's the deeper exhaustion that comes from being pulled in every direction.

When so much of your time, energy and focus is spent looking after others – which women disproportionately do – while managing a demanding career and most likely the lion's share of the housework, it's no wonder there's little left for you. That deep internal spark that makes you want to invest in yourself? It's running on empty.

If you just pile diet and exercise on top of this – two more things on an already overwhelming to-do list – you are setting yourself up for failure. It's most likely why your previous attempts didn't stick. Or why you keep putting it off, waiting for life to get quieter. Spoiler: that time isn't coming. Your life isn't going to get less busy, and it won't be easier to start later. In fact, the longer you leave it, the harder it gets. This is a universal truth for most things we put off.

The real secret to fat loss is to focus on building energy first. Then everything else falls into place. Just like mood, your energy has a baseline – an average level you tend to hover around regardless of what's happening externally. You might get a temporary boost from a holiday or crash after a brutal week, but eventually you return to your set point.

My goal is to help you build your energy baseline. Not so you'll feel 100 per cent every day – that's not realistic. But so that you feel pretty damn good most of the time. Many of my clients tell me their low weeks now are what their good weeks used to feel like. That's the shift we're after.

A higher baseline means more resilience, more motivation and more capacity for the things that matter. You'll still have lower energy days – illness, overwork, poor sleep. But these will be outliers, not the norm.

The Four Pillars

In simple terms, your energy is built on four pillars: sleep, movement, nutrition and stress management. Building your energy starts with identifying which of these is most depleted for you right now, and addressing that first. If your sleep is consistently under six hours, no amount of caffeine or optimistic scheduling will compensate. If your step count is under 3,000 a day, your energy systems are not getting the stimulation they need.

Start with whichever pillar is furthest from where it needs to be – we'll come on to these in the chapters that follow. By that I mean the level your body needs to function at its best. For most people, that looks like around seven to nine hours of sleep, at least 7,000 to 10,000 steps of daily movement, mostly whole-food nutrition in line with your energy needs (not eating too much or too little), and some form of active stress management and life balance – whatever that looks like to you.

The further you are from these targets, the bigger the impact of even small improvements. If you're sleeping four hours, getting to five matters more than going from seven to eight. If you're doing 2,000 steps a day, adding 3,000 has more impact than adding 3,000 on to someone already doing 12,000.

To build your baseline, you don't need to overhaul your entire life overnight. You need to start where you are, focus on the fundamentals and make the adjustments required. And if you're far from your baseline targets, that's not a problem – it's an opportunity to get excited about. You have the most to gain and will likely see the fastest results.

Work With Yourself, Not Against Yourself

Building energy is also about how you think about diet and exercise. If you stop framing diet and exercise as things you *have* to do and start seeing them as things you *get* to do – in order to feel your best and live the life you want – you start to feel like someone who is making choices that are aligned with your goals and values. That shift – from passive victim of circumstance to active agent making deliberate decisions – is one of the most powerful predictors of long-term behaviour change.

In the right dose, diet and exercise give you more energy, not less. When you focus on improving your energy rather than obsessing over weight, calories, macronutrients and step counts, everything else becomes easier. If you still need convincing, just think about the times you've felt genuinely high energy and how much easier it was to make good choices, cook something healthy and say no to things that didn't align with your goals.

So, instead of asking, 'Am I in a deficit today?' start also asking, 'What would give me more energy today?' They're not competing questions. They're complementary ones. And the second one is often easier to answer – and easier to act on. Then, as a byproduct, you make better choices and subsequently end up in a deficit.

I ran this experiment on myself. I had an exceptionally low energy period a few months ago and realised that the way I was living wasn't suited to the way I wanted to feel. So I made a plan and tracked it to hold myself accountable – mood, energy, sleep, food, output – every day for six weeks. The single most impactful change was also the most surprisingly simple one: I did a very short run every day. Under ten minutes. Sometimes just one kilometre. For most people, that sounds like it barely counts or wouldn't be worth doing. But the difference in my mood, my concentration, my resilience to stress and my general capacity to function was significant enough that I've kept doing it ever since.

This is the law of diminishing returns working in your favour. In my experience, you get the vast majority of the benefit from exercise – particularly mood and energy benefits – from the first ten minutes. Which means a ten-minute walk or a one-kilometre run is not a consolation prize for someone who didn't have time to do a proper workout. It is a legitimate, evidence-backed intervention for your mood, your energy and therefore your results.

Can you pick one thing you could do today, in ten minutes or less, that would improve your energy? It might be a short walk. Five minutes outside. A run, a circuit, a glass of water and ten minutes away from your screen. Start there. Remember, energy first. Everything else then follows.

Reframe the stress

Here's a realisation that really helped me: all of your life stress is only stressful because you care. You're stressed about your job because you care about your work. About your partner because the relationship matters to you. About your mortgage because you have a home you want to keep. About your kids because you love them. Every stress is actually something you value.

Seeing it that way allows you to feel grateful for it rather than crushed by it. You don't want anyone to take those stresses away. You want the capacity to handle them. That's what the 'energy-first' approach builds.

Life Fitness

Most people only think about physical fitness in terms of how it looks – abs, a smaller waist, the ability to run a half marathon. But I want to introduce a different concept: life fitness.

Life fitness, at its core, is about capacity. It's your ability to meet the physical and mental demands of your actual life without feeling completely burned out. It's not just about how much you can lift or how many steps your smartwatch says you've done. It's about having energy left in the tank to enjoy your life. Strength for your day. Stamina for your work. Resilience for the hard stuff. Enthusiasm to make the most of the one life you have.

Life fitness gives you the energy to live fully, not just survive. The endurance to get through a stressful week at work, look after the kids and still show up as a partner, friend, sister or grandmother. The mental discipline to keep going when quitting would be easier. The strength to carry your shopping or suitcase, and run for the bus without thinking about it. And, most importantly, to live a healthy, independent, disease-free life for as long as possible. Nothing else matters much if you don't have that.

Exercise is central to this because it increases your energy-generating machinery. Your mitochondria – your internal batteries – multiply and become more efficient in response to consistent training. A 2019 review in *Annual Review of Physiology* found that exercise is the most potent known stimulus for mitochondrial biogenesis – the creation of new mitochondria. Both aerobic exercise and resistance training contribute to this, through different pathways. The practical result: the fitter you become, the more energy you have. Not just for exercise, but for everything. You become fitter not just for the gym, but for life itself.

Energy is the foundation, so fix it first. Everything else – the calorie deficit, the workouts, the nutrition, the consistency – becomes significantly easier when you're not running on empty.

KEY POINTS

- Low energy is the most common reason good intentions don't translate into action. It's not laziness – it's depletion.
- The further you are from your baseline targets, the bigger the return on even small improvements. You have the most to gain.
- Your stresses are actually the things you love. You don't want them gone. You want the capacity to handle them.
- Life fitness is about capacity for your actual life – not a performance metric or an aesthetic.
- Exercise increases mitochondrial density, meaning your body literally becomes more efficient at producing energy. The fitter you are, the more energy you have for everything.

Chapter 15
Decide Once

Let's be honest. Fat loss often feels like a constant battle – a never-ending series of decisions, willpower tests and exhausting mental gymnastics of 'Should I or shouldn't I?' No wonder so many women feel burned out, defeated and stuck in a cycle of starting over.

But what if I told you there's a way to make it easier? A way to free up your mental energy, reduce decision fatigue and build a foundation for lasting results that doesn't require white-knuckling and second-guessing it every single day?

This is the world of automating fat loss. Shifting from relying on fleeting motivation to building habits and systems that make healthy choices your default – not an ongoing battle.

Commit in Advance

I want to be clear: this isn't about being rigid or perfect in execution. It's about being decisive in commitment. My own commitment is to imperfect action in pursuit of my goals. That means I do the best I can in the actual situation I'm in. It means sticking to my Non-Negotiable. Doing the 15-minute workout when I don't have time for a full session. Choosing the best option on a menu even when it's not ideal. Going for a short walk when I know I won't hit my Optimal Target.

That commitment – to always do something rather than nothing, to always make the best available choice rather than waiting for the ideal one, to take the imperfect action rather than waiting for perfect conditions that never come – is what makes it sustainable.

Committing 100 per cent to something also gives you a certain peace. Think about booking travel. You might spend hours weighing up options, comparing prices, deliberating. But once it's booked, it's done. You stop thinking about it. You can apply that same mental liberation to your fat-loss process – but only if you make genuine, clear decisions and then remove the option to negotiate with yourself, because it's that negotiation that is so fatiguing.

The research on deciding in advance

Research on food decision-making backs this up. A 2016 study published in the *Journal of Marketing Research* ran three experiments – two at a corporate cafeteria and one with university students – looking at what happened to food choices depending on how far in advance people ordered their meals. The finding was consistent across all three: the greater the gap between placing the order and eating, the lower the calorie content of what people chose. People who ordered hours ahead consistently chose differently from people who ordered right before eating.

The researchers concluded that decisions made in advance, away from the pull of hunger and the smell of food, draw on a different and more considered part of the brain than decisions made in the moment. Pre-decide your meals and you bypass the version of yourself that is tired, hungry and standing in front of the fridge at 7pm. That version of you is not making your best decisions. The earlier, calmer version of you is.

There is one more dimension to pre-commitment and knowledge of this has shaped many areas of my life. A study of 1,530 Dutch adults measured happiness levels before and after holidays. People who had a holiday booked were significantly happier than those who did not, for weeks before they even left. And once they returned, their happiness levels had dropped back to exactly where they started within a matter of weeks, regardless of how long or enjoyable the trip had been. The conclusion the researchers drew is counterintuitive but consistent with the data: the greatest happiness benefit of a holiday is not the holiday itself. It is having one to look forward to.

This reflects how the human brain processes pleasure. Anticipation – the act of looking forward to something you have committed to – is itself a source of genuine hedonic value (meaning it gives pleasure), distinct from the experience it precedes. Researchers identified this pattern as far back as 1987, showing that people sometimes actively prefer to delay pleasurable experiences – a fancy dinner, a treat they have been looking forward to – because the anticipation adds to the total enjoyment. The waiting is not dead time. It is part of the pleasure.

What makes this especially interesting is a 2017 study that went further still. Across five separate experiments, researchers found that actively savouring an upcoming experience – thinking about it, looking forward to it, engaging with the anticipation rather than just passively waiting – did not just make the waiting more pleasant. It made the actual experience more enjoyable too. People who had spent time anticipating a consumption experience rated it more positively both while it was happening and when they remembered it afterwards. The anticipation created what the researchers called 'affective memory traces' – emotional imprints that were reactivated and integrated into the real experience when it arrived, making the whole experience richer than it would otherwise have been.

Pre-committing to your meals in advance is not just a tool for making better choices. It is also a way of creating something to look forward to. When you decide the night before that tomorrow's dinner is going to be the pad thai you love, or that Friday's meal out is going to be genuinely enjoyed rather than endured with guilt, you are generating anticipatory pleasure that is real and measurable. You are also, according to the research, likely to enjoy the meal itself more when it arrives.

All this is to say that there are numerous upsides to precommitting: you are more likely to follow through, you are more likely to enjoy it and you get a lot of the enjoyment in the anticipation.

Why 100 Per Cent is Easier than 98 Per Cent

This brings us to a concept that changed how I think about consistency, originally from Clayton Christensen: it's easier to hold your principles 100 per cent of the time than 98 per cent of the time. This sounds counterintuitive. Surely 98 per cent gives you more flexibility, more grace, more room? You can argue that, but you can also argue that it tends to lead to constant mental negotiation and decision fatigue – and that is often the most exhausting part of fat loss. Not the diet itself.

The 2 per cent between 98 per cent and 100 per cent is where all the mental anguish lives. It's the space where you constantly have to make choices, negotiate with yourself, re-evaluate and re-commit. Every time. That is exhausting. This continuous internal debate is what psychologists call 'decision fatigue' – and research by Roy Baumeister suggested that willpower and decision-making draw from the same depleting pool. The more decisions you make across the day, the worse your subsequent decisions become. Judges are more likely to grant parole in the morning. Doctors make worse prescribing decisions in the afternoon. Your resolve around food is at its lowest point of the day right when you're most tired, most hungry and most stressed. When you know this, you can work with yourself, not against yourself, by automating decisions and committing to them 100 per cent.

Think about a lifelong vegetarian. Do they wake up every day and consciously decide not to eat meat? No. They made that decision once and it's simply who they are now. The decision is automated. They don't spend mental energy debating whether to have a beef burger – it's not even an option. It's far easier to be 100 per cent meat-free than 98 per cent meat-free, because the 2 per cent requires constant vigilance, constant re-evaluation, and constant willpower and decision-making expenditure.

The same principle applies to any dietary commitment. If you've decided you don't eat breakfast before noon, you don't spend your morning debating breakfast. The decision is made. The mental energy is preserved for everything else.

It's important to say here that you should be selective about what you commit to – not everything deserves a 100 per cent commitment. But once you've decided, commit fully. Pair this with what you learned about range targets in Chapter 5 and genuinely watch your life and your results change. Stop wasting energy on constant deliberation. Decide what standards you hold. Set range targets around them and commit to them fully. Automate those behaviours and watch the results arrive as a natural by-product of the life you've built.

In Chapter 18, I explain the framework I have created to do this around your food choices. It's how I manage to stay lean with minimal effort. I also do a small amount of exercise/movement every morning and it takes almost no effort to do so because it's just what I do. It's ingrained, it's easy and I made that decision years ago and simply stuck to it. I don't decide to do it every day. I decided once – and I think that is the gap between seeing someone who is consistent and wondering how on earth they do it, and realising they are doing it somewhat effortlessly.

From Commitment to Autopilot

Habits are how 100 per cent commitments become automatic. James Clear describes the habit loop elegantly in *Atomic Habits*: cue → craving → response → reward. A trigger initiates the behaviour. A craving motivates it. The response is the habit itself. The reward reinforces it.

When you commit 100 per cent to a new habit, you're working to make the response automatic – bypassing the need for willpower to initiate it each time. The goal is for your brain to stop treating it as a decision and start treating it as simply what you do. 'I go for a walk after dinner' is not a decision I make each evening. It's just what happens after dinner.

To build habits that stick, James Clear's four laws are the most practical framework I've found. But I want to show you exactly what they look like in practice:

1. **Make the behaviour obvious.** The habit has to be visible and pre-decided, otherwise your tired evening brain will talk you out of it. I lay out my workout clothes the night before. Removing that one decision removes the excuse. With clients, I use what I call the 'friction audit': we go through their day and make the good decisions as easy and frictionless as possible – the choice you want to make should be the easy choice. Nobody is strong enough to out-willpower their environment at 9pm after a long stressful day and poor sleep. So we change the environment instead to set yourself up for success.
2. **Make it attractive.** I only listen to one particular podcast when I'm running. Not at any other time. Running. Only. It means I actually look forward to going. With clients, the equivalent is often a playlist they only play during workouts, or a coffee they have on training mornings. You're borrowing motivation from something you already enjoy and attaching it to something you're building. Reward yourself, make it enjoyable. Bonus here: the easiest way to make

workouts easier is to do is with a friend. It takes less than half the motivation!

3. **Make it easy.** Start smaller than feels necessary. I mean this literally. One client – a busy GP with two young children – couldn't sustain any workout routine for longer than 30 minutes. Every plan she'd ever tried had fallen apart within weeks. We dropped it to 20 minutes, three times a week. She's been consistent for seven months. A 20-minute session you do beats a 60-minute session you skip.
4. **Make it satisfying.** Tick something off. There is a reason I ask clients to track their workouts – not only do I want to see it, but it also produces a small but real dopamine response that reinforces the loop. You're teaching your brain that this behaviour feels good. Over time, the behaviour becomes its own reward. Until then, manufacture the satisfaction: track your streak, note how you feel after training, celebrate the fact that you showed up.

Automating fat loss is not about a quick fix or a temporary phase. It's about building a way of living – eating, moving, sleeping, managing stress – that you can repeat indefinitely without burning out. One you actually enjoy and that supports your energy, your health and the life you want.

Build a life where the right choice is the one that requires minimal thought. Automate your decisions and then watch what becomes possible while you get on with living your life and let your choices compound.

KEY POINTS

- The 2 per cent between 98 per cent and 100 per cent is where all the mental anguish lives. A 100 per cent commitment removes the need to negotiate with yourself every single time.
- Decision fatigue is real: willpower depletes across the day. The goal is to remove as many food and exercise decisions as possible so your limited willpower stays reserved for things that actually require it.
- A 100 per cent commitment means decisive commitment to imperfect action – always doing something rather than nothing, always choosing the best available option rather than waiting for perfect conditions.
- Building strong habits means making the right response automatic, bypassing willpower entirely: cue → craving → response → reward.

Chapter 16

Making Your Bad Days Less Bad

In Chapter 5, we talked about range targets and how they free you from the all-or-nothing cycle. We established that real, lasting fat loss doesn't come from hitting the bullseye every single day – it comes from consistently staying on the board. Now, let's get practical about how you actually do that on the days when everything feels hard.

Making your bad days less bad is the single most impactful strategy you can adopt for sustainable fat loss. Not making your good days more extreme. Not finding a better diet. Not training harder when motivation is high. But managing what happens when it isn't.

The Snakes and Ladders Problem

Most people approach fat loss like snakes and ladders. They're either landing on ladders – perfect days, great choices, everything aligned – or they're hitting snakes and sliding all the way back to the start. A few good days, one bad one, and they're not just paused, they're behind where they started, often significantly.

This is exhausting. Three steps forward, two and a half steps back. Net progress is minimal. You're expending enormous effort for almost no return, which is demoralising and – understandably – leads to giving up entirely.

But it's so important to remember that your current body composition is a reflection of your average energy balance *over time*. Not that one perfect week. Not that one disastrous weekend. The sum total of all your choices, consistently applied over months and years. And the biggest impact you have on that average isn't making your good days more perfect, it's making your bad days less bad.

What This Looks Like in Practice

Example one: workouts. Let's say you're aiming for five a week. Life happens – a sick child, work deadline, genuine exhaustion. In the all-or-nothing mindset, if you can't do five, there's no point doing any. You go from five to zero. In the 'less bad' approach, your Non-Negotiable is three. If five isn't possible this week, three is. You still end the week closer to your goals than you started.

Example two: calories. Say your Optimal Target is 1,500 and your Non-Negotiable is 2,000. You have a stressful day, eat lunch with friends and end up at 1,800. All-or-nothing says the day is blown, might as well finish the evening with everything in the kitchen. Range target thinking says: 1,800 is still under my 2,000 Non-Negotiable. Still a deficit. Still moving forward. Take the win.

Example three: steps. Imagine your Optimal is 12,000 and your Non-Negotiable is 7,000. You have a busy day of back-to-back meetings. Instead of accepting 3,000 steps, you take a 15-minute walk at lunch, pace during phone calls and park further from the entrance. You hit 7,000. On a day that felt awful, you still moved forward.

The choice to hit your minimum on a difficult day is far more powerful than trying to add extra on an already good day. It prevents you going backwards. It keeps your average moving in the right direction. And over weeks and months, that really adds up.

The Investing Analogy

Think of your fat-loss journey like long-term investing. You wouldn't expect to get rich by making one enormous investment and then losing everything on the next. Wealth is built through consistent, smart decisions over time – even when some days the market is down. That is an opportunity to make better returns. Making your bad days less bad is where the biggest opportunity is.

Your fat loss works the same way. The dramatic swings – perfect days followed by complete collapses – cancel each other out. The investor who slowly, steadily adds to their portfolio without ever having a catastrophic loss outperforms the one who swings wildly every time. Boring consistency beats exciting volatility, every time.

The Non-Negotiable on your bad days is your protection against the catastrophic loss. It keeps you in the game. It means that even your worst weeks are still weeks of forward progress.

Motivation Is Not the Answer

Many people wait for motivation before they act: 'Once I feel motivated, I'll start eating properly and exercising.' But motivation is a *consequence* of action, not a precondition for it. It comes after you start, not before. And it's not reliable enough to build a strategy around.

This is where making bad days less bad becomes essential. It's not about motivation. It's about having a pre-decided plan for the days when motivation is absent.

The if-then plan

As we saw in the previous chapter, the principle behind pre-commitment is straightforward: decisions made in advance, in a calm and rational state, are almost always better than decisions made in the moment, when you're tired, hungry or stressed. The if-then plan is one of the most studied and effective forms of pre-commitment available and it is very powerful. Psychologist Peter Gollwitzer, who has spent decades researching what he calls 'implementation intentions', found that simply deciding in advance *when, where and how* you will do something more than doubles the likelihood that you'll actually do it – across hundreds of studies, in contexts ranging from exercise to diet to medication adherence. It's not about motivation. It's about removing the in-the-moment decision entirely. It's about making a commitment to yourself that you honour, regardless of how you feel – within realistic limits that account for actual human variation.

Here's how it works: decide in advance how you'll respond to specific situations. For example:

- 'If it's Monday morning, then I go to the gym.'
- 'If I'm offered something that doesn't help me with my goals and doesn't excite me either, then I politely decline.'
- 'If I get home late and haven't got anything in for dinner then I order the pho because I know it's a healthy and fast option.'
- 'If I'm having a bad day, then I aim for my Non-Negotiable rather than my Optimal. But I always make sure I am moving forward in the direction of my goal each day.'

Pre-decided responses eliminate the in-the-moment negotiation that low mood or decision fatigue always win.

This isn't about striving for perfection or accepting mediocrity. It's about understanding that life is genuinely messy, and building a system that works within that reality. Bad days are not obstacles to your fat-loss journey. They're part of it. The goal is not to eliminate them – it's to minimise their impact and never let them become a reason to stop.

Anyone can stay consistent when motivation is high and life is smooth. The real work happens on hard days. That's where results are actually built.

KEY POINTS

- Your body composition reflects your average energy balance over time, not your best days or your worst ones. The average is what matters.

- Three steps forward and two and a half steps back produces minimal net progress despite enormous effort. Three steps forward and then one step forward on bad days alters the entire trajectory.
- The minimum effective dose on a difficult day beats zero every time. It's not settling for less – it's protecting your average.
- Motivation follows action – it doesn't precede it. Having a pre-decided plan for low-motivation days removes the need to 'feel like it' before starting.
- Self-trust is built by keeping commitments on hard days. That evidence changes your belief about what you're capable of sustaining.
- If-then planning pre-decides responses to common situations, eliminating in-the-moment negotiation. Decide in advance – then just execute.

Chapter 17

Protein: The One Thing That Actually Earns Its Place

I spent Part 2 telling you that most of what the fitness industry sells you is unnecessary. So let me tell you about the one thing that isn't.

If there is a single dietary factor that has more impact on fat loss, muscle retention, hunger management and long-term metabolic health than any other, it's protein. Not a supplement. Not a protocol. Not a carefully timed eating window. Just protein. Consistently, every single day. And yet most women aren't eating enough of it.

In this chapter, I want to explain why it matters so much, how much you actually need and why it's genuinely harder for women to get there than most nutrition advice acknowledges.

What Protein Actually Does

Most people think of protein as the thing that builds muscle. And it does – but that's the smallest part of why it matters for fat loss.

Protein is the most satiating macronutrient. Gram for gram,

it keeps you fuller for longer than carbohydrates or fat. This happens in three ways:

1. It triggers the release of cholecystokinin (CCK) and peptide YY (PYY) – the gut peptide hormones that signal fullness.
2. It suppresses ghrelin – the hormone that drives hunger.
3. It slows gastric emptying, meaning food stays in your stomach longer.

It also has the highest thermic effect (see page 13) of the three macronutrients (carbohydrates, protein and fat). Your body burns approximately 20–30 per cent of protein's calories just through the process of digesting it. For carbohydrates, that figure is 5–10 per cent. For fat, it's 0–3 per cent. This means that 100 calories of protein effectively delivers around 70–80 net calories. Not a massive difference on its own, but across a whole day of eating it adds up. Studies consistently show that people who eat adequate protein during a calorie deficit lose more fat and retain more muscle than those eating the same calories with less protein.

And then there's muscle preservation. When you're in a calorie deficit, your body needs energy from somewhere. If you're not eating enough protein and resistance training, a larger portion of that energy will come from breaking down muscle tissue – not just fat. This matters for three reasons. First, muscle is a metabolically active tissue – losing it lowers your BMR, making it harder to maintain fat loss over time. Second, the look and feel so many people are after – strong, lean, defined – comes from having muscle, not just losing weight. Third, and most importantly, muscle is really, really important for health. Having more muscle mass improves your metabolic health and lowers your risk of chronic diseases.

How Much Do You Actually Need?

The official UK recommended intake for protein is 0.75g per kilogram of body weight per day. For a 70kg woman, that's about 52g. Across a day, that might look like: two eggs at breakfast (~12g), a tuna sandwich at lunch (~20g) and a portion of chicken or salmon at dinner (~20g). That is the minimum required to prevent deficiency in a sedentary person. It is not the target for a woman who is trying to lose fat, maintain muscle and support her long-term health.

The research on optimal protein for fat loss and body composition is considerably more generous. Most sports nutrition guidelines and fat loss research suggest a target of 1.6–2.2g per kilogram of body weight per day for people who are training and trying to change their body composition. For a 70kg woman, that's 112–154g of protein per day.

To put those numbers in context: a chicken breast contains roughly 30–35g of protein. A large egg contains about 6g. A tin of tuna contains 25g. A portion of Greek yoghurt contains 10–15g. Getting to 120g a day requires deliberate, consistent effort. For most women, it means actively building protein into every meal rather than treating it as an afterthought.

It's important to note that there are diminishing returns above roughly 100–140g for most women. The satiety benefits don't continue to climb indefinitely and, above that range, you're displacing other foods in your diet without proportional benefit.

The goal isn't maximum protein – it's consistent, adequate protein.

Why Women Specifically Struggle with This

There are a few reasons why protein tends to be lower in women's diets, and they're worth understanding rather than just being told to 'eat more protein'.

First, many women have spent years in diet culture environments that demonised fat and then carbohydrates, but never once talked about getting enough protein. The legacy of low-fat dieting in particular – where yoghurts, cereals and crackers were marketed as healthy because they were low in fat but were often low in protein and high in refined carbs – left a generation of women eating meals that were suboptimal. Protein was just ignored.

Second, the most protein-dense foods – meat, fish, eggs, dairy – are also the foods that diet culture has most complicated. Years of messaging about red meat being bad, eggs raising cholesterol and dairy being inflammatory have made many women genuinely uncertain about whether these foods are okay to eat. The anxiety around them is real, even if most of it isn't warranted by current evidence.

And finally, there's the social dynamics around food. Women are more likely to eat smaller portions at social occasions, more likely to have their eating habits noticed and commented on, and historically more likely to have had their dietary choices shaped by what's considered 'appropriate' rather than what's optimal: for example, women should be full after a small salad and not order the steak. I hope you're rolling your eyes reading this. The tide is changing slightly but we are not there yet.

The Practical Side

Getting to adequate protein doesn't require eating chicken and broccoli at every meal. It requires building a framework and sticking to it.

The simplest approach I use with clients is the protein-first rule: at every meal, decide what your protein source is before anything else. Not 'I'll have pasta with some chicken on top', but 'I'll have chicken, and I'll build the rest of the meal around it'. The protein is the anchor. Everything else is the side.

Good protein sources include:

- chicken
- turkey
- beef
- pork
- fish
- shellfish
- eggs
- Greek yoghurt
- cottage cheese
- low-fat soft cheese
- tofu
- tempeh
- edamame
- legumes (beans, lentils, chickpeas)
- protein powder if needed (more on this below)

A practical daily structure that works for most women is:

- 30–40g of protein at breakfast (eggs, Greek yoghurt, protein shake if needed – not all together of course; take your pick)
- 40–50g at lunch (chicken, fish or legume-based)
- 40–50g at dinner (lean meat or fish)
- small protein contributions from snacks (a small pot of cottage cheese (12g), an edamame snack (9g) or half a tin of tuna (16g) – these small amounts add up and make hitting your daily target much more manageable)

That gets most people to 120g without precision tracking. (See page 271 for more detail on portion sizes and protein amounts in other common foods.)

Protein powder becomes relevant when you're consistently struggling to hit your protein target from whole food alone, which is genuinely difficult for many women in a calorie deficit. If you want to supplement with protein powder – I often do – then whey protein has the best leucine content (the amino acid most important for muscle protein synthesis) and mixes well. For vegans or vegetarians, a soya or pea-and-rice blend is a good alternative. Look for products with at least 20g of protein per serving and minimal added sugar.

A note on plant-based protein: it's absolutely possible to hit adequate protein on a plant-based diet, but it requires more planning because most plant proteins are less bioavailable (i.e. your body absorbs a smaller percentage) and come packaged with more carbohydrates and calories. Tofu, tempeh, edamame, seitan and protein supplements are the most efficient plant-based options. Relying on beans and lentils alone makes the maths much harder.

One of the easier nutritional principles to implement is to simply build each meal around protein. Do that consistently and you will naturally eat less overall, recover better from training and hold on to more muscle during your deficit.

KEY POINTS

- Protein is the most satiating macronutrient and has the highest thermic effect of food. It suppresses ghrelin, triggers CCK and PYY, and slows gastric emptying.
- The UK recommended intake of 0.75g per kg of body weight is a minimum for sedentary people. For fat loss and muscle retention, aim for 1.6–2.2g per kg.
- Protein-first thinking: decide your protein source before building the rest of the meal. It's the anchor, not the afterthought.
- The muscle you build and maintain now is the muscle that keeps your metabolism healthy, your bones strong and your body functional for decades.

Chapter 18

The 3:1 Method

I've been coaching women for over 15 years and, in that time, I've tried, tested and observed dozens of different dietary approaches. Most of them work in principle. Very few of them work in practice, long-term, for real women with real lives.

The 3:1 method is the exception. It's the single most practical fat-loss framework I've ever used with clients, and it's the one I come back to again and again – because it fits the way most women actually live. It's simple enough to become automatic. Flexible enough to include a social life. And it works.

I've described this method as one of the most simple and effective strategies to lose fat in an enjoyable way. Having used it with thousands of clients, I stand by that. This is also the framework I use for my own nutrition. However, this is just one way to structure your eating day and, in my experience, it works well for most people, but it is not the only way to eat. This is not a diet book, remember. However, I have a rule where if I am going to try anything, I stick to it for 30 days before I decide if it's working or not. Deciding something isn't working after a week is not a good test. Please give yourself time and the same minimum commitment when it comes to this method.

The Premise

The 3:1 method is straightforward: you structure your eating day in two distinct phases:

- Three consistent, pre-planned, nutrient-dense meals during the day: breakfast, lunch and a snack.
- More flexibility for dinner in the evening.

The first three meals stay largely the same day to day. They're built around whole foods, protein and hitting your fruit and vegetable intake. As health-focused as possible. These aren't necessarily designed to be exciting meals. They're not supposed to be. They're your foundation and are built for function while you're busy living life.

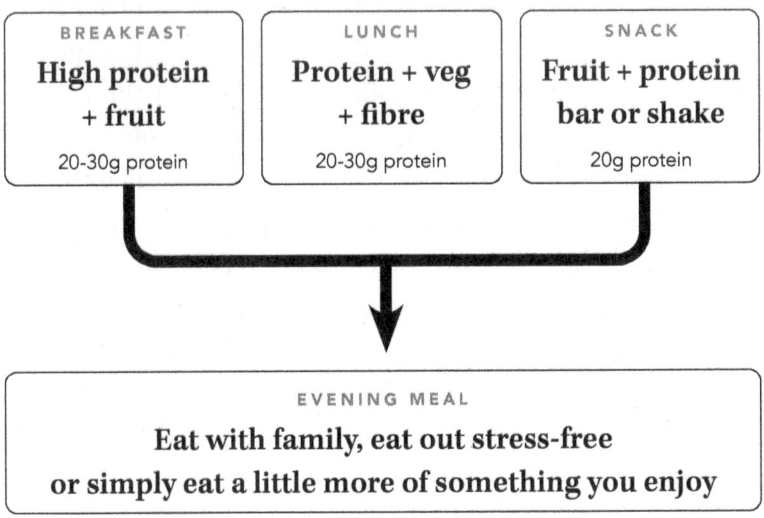

The 3:1 method

When I say 'whole foods', what I mean is simply foods that are as close to their natural state as possible: think chicken breast, eggs, oats, rice, potatoes, lentils, fruit, vegetables and nuts. Whole foods are foods that don't have an ingredients list, or have one short enough that you could have made it yourself. The opposite is ultra-processed food – products that have been heavily manufactured, often stripped of nutrients and loaded with additives to make them more palatable and shelf-stable. This isn't about being puritanical. The occasional biscuit is not going to derail you. But a diet built predominantly on whole foods will keep you fuller for longer, provide more micronutrients per calorie, support your energy levels and make hitting your protein and fibre targets significantly easier. It's not complicated. It's just food that actually does something useful.

When it comes to fruit and vegetables, the target most commonly cited in the research – and the one the NHS recommends – is five portions a day, where a portion is roughly 80g. That's the minimum worth aiming for, not the ceiling. Studies consistently show that risk of cardiovascular disease, type 2 diabetes and several cancers continues to fall as intake increases up to around seven to ten portions per day. Practically, aim to have at least one portion of fruit or vegetables with every main meal, and use your snack to add another. Variety matters, too – different colours provide different phytonutrients, so a plate that looks colourful is usually doing more work than one that doesn't. If hitting five feels difficult right now, start there. But know that more is genuinely better.

By the end of those three meals, you've hit three solid servings of protein at roughly 20–30g each. You've nailed your five portions of fruit and vegetables. You've eaten real, nourishing food. And depending on your specific choices, you're sitting at somewhere around 1,100 calories – leaving you with 500–800 calories of flexibility for the evening, if your Optimal Target is around 1,600–1,900.

That flexibility is the whole point. The evening meal is usually where you live your life – eating with your family, going out for dinner, having a glass of wine, having the time to cook something you actually enjoy and having something to look forward to at the end of the day. The 3:1 method doesn't require you to eat diet food at the dinner table or be the person at the restaurant quietly calculating macros while everyone else orders normally. You've done the work during the day, so the evening can be more flexible.

This is just an example. You can mould the framework to suit you, your needs, your life, your goals, your constraints and how you like eating. The key to it is that you have structure, but not so much structure that it feels rigid and unsustainable.

In Chapter 15, we talked about decision fatigue – the way that every decision you make draws from the same limited mental resource, so that by evening your resolve is at its lowest point precisely when temptation is typically highest. The 3:1 method is, in large part, a solution to this problem. Once you know what your food structure and choices are for the day, it's much easier to tick the boxes and get on with using your valuable brain power for more important things, as you're not making those decisions from scratch every morning or every mealtime.

By keeping your first three meals largely consistent, you make the decision once – not every single day. You decide what your breakfast looks like, what your lunch looks like and what your snack looks like. You don't need to eat the exact same thing every day – the goal is to have a small rotation of options for each meal slot so you're not deciding from scratch every time you're hungry. It's about variety within a consistent structure, rather than total spontaneity. Mix up your fruit and veg options, and ideally eat what is in season. There's no thinking involved, no willpower required, no standing in front of the fridge at 7am trying to figure out what to eat while also answering emails. The less you have to decide, the more consistent you are and the less you overthink.

This is exactly what Chapter 15 described: reducing the friction, removing the decision and making the healthy choice the default. The 3:1 method is that principle applied directly to your daily eating structure.

The 3:1 Method Is Designed for Real Life

Most dietary approaches fail in the evening. Not because people have no willpower after 6pm, but because any eating approach that can't accommodate the evenings when 'life' tends to happen is an eating approach you'll abandon because it feels like you're missing out. And let's be real, you are. There is only so long you will put up with missing out without becoming resentful.

The 3:1 method is built around the reality of how most of the women I work with actually live and offers the perfect balance between structure and flexibility: structure during the day, when there's a routine to follow, decisions are easier and you rarely have time to sit and enjoy food anyway because you're working or rushing around after the kids; flexibility in the evening, when social eating happens and rigid rules create friction, guilt, resentment and the all-or-nothing spiral.

There's also a satiety argument here. By the time evening comes, you've already eaten two protein-rich, high-fibre, high-volume meals and one snack. Your ghrelin is lower, your fullness hormones are better regulated and you're not arriving at dinner ravenous and likely to overeat – you're arriving hungry and looking forward to a nice meal, but in control. That makes the flexible evening meal much easier to enjoy without overdoing it.

And because the evening meal is flexible – not a carefully measured exception, but actual freedom to eat what you want within a reasonable range – it doesn't feel like a diet at all. By 'reasonable range', I mean a sensible estimate of the calories within your evening meal that would still align with your calorie range targets for the day. This is not permission to eat whatever you like: the range is deliberate and still creates a consistent deficit. It simply removes the all-or-nothing pressure and perceived restriction that causes most people to give up. But I want to be real here, and also my editor told me to add this: if you stick to the 3:1 method but then overeat in the evening meal and kid yourself you are in a deficit, guess what? You won't lose fat. But when you do this right – when you own your food choices, when you see them as empowered and goal-driven because you want to feel your best and those choices are in line with that outcome – it feels like self-care, because it is.

The reason I created the 3:1 method was because it's how I was eating, staying lean and living myself but without really conceptualising it. The beauty is, you don't need to tell anyone you're on a diet or trying to lose fat. You eat the same dinner as everyone else. You order from the same restaurant menu. You're just someone who eats well during the day and sensibly in the evening by choosing your indulgences and enjoying them when it matters. But – and this is the point I want to be clear on – you have to *own* those choices. You won't get results from the work you didn't do or from the good choices you didn't make.

Getting Started with the 3:1 Method

The hardest part of any new approach is the first week, when it is not automatic yet. The good news is, it's only a week and then it gets a lot easier.

Here is a simple way to begin.

Start by deciding what your three daytime meals will look like. They do not need to be exciting – they need to be repeatable. Choose a high-protein breakfast you genuinely enjoy eating most mornings, a lunch that you can prepare quickly or buy reliably, and a mid-afternoon snack built around protein and fruit. Write them down. These are your defaults.

It might look something like:

- Breakfast: Fresh berries and high-protein yoghurt
- Lunch: Chicken salad with pita bread
- Snack: Protein bar and mango

This is my go-to most days – I rotate the salad options and fruit choices, but keep the same basic structure so I can get on with my busy life. Then, in the evening, when I am more likely to eat socially or have time to sit down and enjoy my meal, I have something I fancy.

Here are some other ideas:

- Breakfast: Scrambled eggs with spinach and a piece of fruit

- Lunch: Soup with chicken or a plant-based protein, and roast vegetables
- Snack: Cottage cheese with cucumber and cherry tomatoes
- Breakfast: Overnight oats with protein powder, berries and a handful of nuts
- Lunch: Big salad bowl with salmon or chickpeas, roasted peppers, spinach, quinoa and a tahini dressing
- Snack: Apple with peanut butter and a boiled egg
- Breakfast: Smoked salmon and eggs on rye bread
- Lunch: Grilled chicken or tuna salad with mixed leaves, cucumber, cherry tomatoes and a boiled egg
- Snack: High-protein yoghurt with a banana

A plant-based day might look like:

- Breakfast: Tofu scramble with peppers and a piece of fruit
- Lunch: Lentil and roasted vegetable soup with a side of Greek yoghurt or a small portion of feta
- Snack: Edamame and a handful of mixed berries

Each example hits roughly 20–30g of protein per meal, contributes at least three of the five fruit and veg portions, and lands in the 900–1,200 calorie range. I've given a few examples here, but I would stick with fewer options to reduce decision fatigue.

Track your three meals properly just once – weigh portions and log everything accurately – so you know exactly what you are eating and can verify that you are hitting your protein and staying within your calorie range targets. After that first thorough tracking session, you do not need to track them again. You already know. That is the magic of consistent meals. You don't need to stress over little changes to salad, veg or fruit, but you do need a basic awareness of calorie content – so it is worth knowing, for example, that adding avocado to a salad instead of cucumber is going to bump up the calories due to the fat content or that swapping potato for rice is going to add calories if you are not adjusting portion sizes. This is why tracking initially is important, so you have a baseline understanding.

For the evening meal, set a simple calorie range rather than a fixed number. If your range target is 1,600–1,900 calories for fat loss and your three daytime meals come to around 1,100, your evening range is 500–800 calories. That gives you real flexibility. A home-cooked meal, a restaurant dinner or an evening with a glass of wine and something simple – all of it fits. Of course, it's also important to adjust as you go. If you find your daytime meals are leaving you too hungry by evening, add more fibre and protein. There should also be a focus on keeping food volume high when dieting – more on this in Chapter 21.

The 3:1 method is a structure, not a rigid prescription. Mould it to your life and it will work. Most of my clients settle into their version of it within two weeks and describe it as the first eating approach that has ever felt genuinely sustainable and like they are not even on a diet.

The Tracking Problem

One of the things I hear most from women starting out with calorie tracking is that it becomes all-consuming. They spend more time logging food than enjoying it. They get anxious when they can't find the exact item in the app or when someone else has cooked dinner for them. They feel like failures if the numbers don't add up perfectly and so end up thinking 'screw it'.

I built the 3:1 method as a solution to this. Rather than constantly being on your phone and trying to track everything, you simply track your three structured daytime meals once. Just once. Get a clear picture of roughly what you're eating – the portion sizes, the protein content, the rough calorie range, the fibre – then, because these meals stay largely the same, you don't need to track them again. You already know.

For the evening meal, use a rough estimate within your remaining calorie range. You don't need to weigh your pasta to the gram. You need a reasonable ballpark. People get ridiculously analytical about calorie tracking, spending hours agonising over numbers that are, by the nature of the system, already an approximation. Even if you're very good at tracking accurately, which most people are not, food database entries are imprecise. Cooking changes calorie content. Portion sizes vary. The caloric availability of food varies. And so being consistent and making adjustments based on progress matters far more than achieving a precise daily number because that precise number really isn't all that precise.

Track once to understand your baseline. Then use that understanding to guide sensible choices, rather than turning every meal into a data entry exercise.

Who This Works Best For

The 3:1 method works particularly well for women with social lives, careers and families – which is to say, most of the women

I work with. If your days have some structure and your evenings vary, this maps onto your life naturally. The consistency happens when consistency is easy, i.e. when you are busy through the day. The flexibility happens when you actually need it, i.e. when you want to eat socially in the evening.

It also works well for anyone who finds constant tracking overwhelming or unsustainable, or who has struggled with all-or-nothing thinking around food. Because the three daytime meals are decided in advance and largely habitual, there's very little to slip up on during the day. And because the evening is genuinely flexible, there's nothing to 'cheat' on or feel guilty about. This is how you lose fat without feeling restricted or like you're missing out. And that is essential if you want to maintain it.

The 3:1 method is easily adaptable to those whose days are highly unpredictable too – shift workers, frequent travellers or people who love brunch on the weekend (me). For those situations, the framework may need adapting, but the underlying principle – applying structure to your nutrition and decisions around food and banking some extra calories for the meal where you want more flexibility – applies regardless of which meal that ends up being.

If there's one thing I want you to take from this chapter, it's this: sustainability comes from building an approach that fits your actual life, not from finding a diet you can endure for a fixed period. The 3:1 method fits real life. That's why it works.

There are also some extra unexpected benefits you get from the 3:1 method. The biggest for me personally being productivity. I find I am far more productive when I am not debating what I might have for breakfast or lunch and also when I am structured so I am fuelling myself well. It means I can focus my finite brain power where it's best used – coaching clients and building my business, not thinking about food constantly.

If you also decide to pre-prepare your meals and buy food for the week rather than daily, you will save money with this method too. Planning and preparing becomes a lot easier when you know what you are eating for 75 per cent of the day. The alternative is usually to nip into a supermarket or coffee shop for a quick snack or lunch option. This really adds up over the week (it is somehow impossible to go into a supermarket and not spend at least £10 even when you're going in for one thing).

Using the 3:1 method will make you leaner, more focused and wealthier all in one. That's a pretty great outcome, if you ask me!

Just a reminder here: I've shown you how many of my clients – and myself – structure their eating by using the 3:1 method. You can choose to use this or not, but the key principle is having a structure of eating that works for you, allows you to eat in line with your energy needs without restriction and gives you the flexibility to enjoy life while staying in shape. You learned the key principles of energy balance in Chapter 1, so find a way in which you can fit that into your life. If the 3:1 method doesn't work for you or needs tweaking, give yourself the flexibility to do that.

You make the decision about your daytime meals once. Then you just execute. No willpower required, no thinking involved, no daily negotiation with yourself. That's the whole point. Then you get to use your brain power for more important things.

KEY POINTS

- The 3:1 method consists of: three consistent, protein-rich, whole-food meals during the day, leaving 600–800 calories of flexibility for the evening meal.
- By keeping daytime meals consistent, you make the decision once rather than repeatedly under pressure. This directly reduces decision fatigue.
- Front-loading nutrition means arriving at the evening meal with hunger hormones better regulated – in control rather than ravenous.
- Track your three daytime meals once to understand your baseline. After that, consistency matters more than daily precision.

Chapter 19

Exercise: The Magic Pill

If exercise were a drug, it would be the most remarkable thing ever discovered. Doctors would prescribe it for depression, anxiety, type 2 diabetes, cardiovascular disease, osteoporosis, certain cancers, dementia and about 50 other conditions. It would be on the front page of every newspaper. It would be the most talked-about medical breakthrough of our lifetimes.

The problem is that we've spent decades reducing exercise to a calorie-burning tool. We've turned movement into punishment for eating, a chore to earn your dinner, a counter on a treadmill. We've stripped out everything that makes it extraordinary and left women thinking about it purely in terms of what it does to their body size. I want to change that framing entirely. Not because weight and body composition don't matter; they do. But because if you only see exercise through the lens of fat loss, you're missing the majority of its value.

Exercise is not just a non-negotiable for fat loss – in fact, it's not really for fat loss at all because, as we touched on in Chapter 1, the impact of exercise on fat loss is much smaller than most people think – but for health, mood, energy and long-term independence. If you're not strength training, you're leaving the most important factor for long-term health out. And if you're not moving enough across the day, your metabolic health will suffer.

Fitness Versus Body Size

Before anything else, I want to address a misconception that informs how most women think about exercise. We tend to assume that body size tells us everything about health: a smaller body means healthy; a larger body means unhealthy. But the research tells a very different story.

Fitness, specifically cardiovascular fitness, is a significantly better predictor of health and longevity than body mass index (BMI – a measure of weight relative to height) or body fat percentage. Studies consistently show that people who are 'fit and obese' have dramatically lower health risks than people who are inactive and lean. Low physical fitness has a bigger impact on mortality than obesity does.

I want to be clear here: I'm not saying that weight doesn't matter or that excess body fat has no health consequences. It does. Being lean and fit is healthier than being overweight and fit. But fitness is a better predictor of health outcomes than body fat, and that distinction has important implications for how you think about exercise.

If you've recently increased your exercise and the scales haven't moved yet, please do not give up. You are doing yourself an enormous amount of good. Your cardiovascular health, your metabolic function, your mental well-being, your bone density and your long-term independence are all improving, even if your jeans fit the same. Health is not a size. Fitness is one of its most powerful pillars.

A note on NEAT (see page 12) here: a fascinating study by James Levine at the Mayo Clinic found that lean individuals tend to stand and move casually for around two and a half hours more per day than obese individuals. Not from deliberate exercise, just from the small unconscious movements that make up a day. His research suggests that this difference alone could account for around 350 calories per day. The implication: your daily step count and general fidgeting matter.

The good news is that NEAT is almost infinitely flexible. You don't need to schedule it, kit up for it or recover from it. You just need to nudge it upwards – consistently, across the whole day. Here's how to do that in practice:

- **Set a movement minimum, not just a step target.** Rather than aiming for 10,000 steps as an abstract number, identify your current daily average and add 2,000–3,000 steps to it. That's your new minimum Non-Negotiable, regardless of whether you trained that day. Most people find this more achievable than a fixed target that bears no relation to where they're starting from. Note: there is a ceiling here – if you are getting around 10,000–12,000 steps daily, adding more is not necessarily better and can increase hunger.
- **Use your phone against itself.** Every time you take or make a phone call, stand up and walk. This alone adds meaningful movement to most people's days without requiring a single extra decision.

- **Rethink your defaults.** Park further away as a rule, not occasionally. Take the stairs. Walk to a colleague's desk instead of emailing. Eat lunch away from your desk. None of these things feel like exercise because they aren't – and that's the point. NEAT works through accumulation, not intensity.
- **Use a stand-up prompt.** If you work at a desk, set a recurring reminder every hour to stand and move around for five minutes. Five minutes per hour across an eight-hour workday is 40 minutes of additional low-level movement that costs you nothing in time or effort. You will find you are more productive too.
- **Walk after meals.** Even for ten minutes. Walking after eating improves blood glucose management, contributes to your daily step count and – as a bonus – often helps digestion too.

What Exercise Actually Does to Your Body

When researchers look at exercise and all-cause mortality (meaning death from any cause, used in research as the most comprehensive measure of a health intervention's overall impact), the results are remarkably consistent. Physically active people live longer. Not just because they avoid one specific disease, but because movement reduces the risk of dying from cardiovascular disease, cancer, metabolic conditions and neurodegenerative diseases, all at the same time.

The biggest health gains come from moving from being completely inactive to doing something. That first step is the most powerful one. You don't need to be training for a marathon or lifting heavy weights to get a significant health benefit. You need to not be sedentary.

If you are starting from zero, no problem. Here is your first step: go for a 20-minute walk. Just a walk. Outside if possible, because the evidence for natural light and mood is solid and fresh air costs nothing. Twenty minutes. Today. This is not a placeholder until you start 'properly'. The research on sedentary behaviour is clear that the transition from inactive to lightly active produces significant health benefits.

Regular exercise strengthens your heart and improves vascular function – the health and efficiency of your blood vessels, which affects blood pressure, circulation and your long-term risk of heart disease and stroke. It enhances insulin sensitivity, which is protective against type 2 diabetes. It improves immune surveillance – the immune system's ongoing process of surveying the body for abnormal cells, which is one of the mechanisms by which regular exercise is thought to reduce cancer risk. It increases brain-derived neurotrophic factor, a protein which supports the growth of new neurons and is one of the reasons exercise is so powerfully protective against depression and dementia. It maintains bone density. It improves sleep quality. And it reduces chronic inflammation.

There is no drug that does all of these things simultaneously with so few downsides. None. Exercise is the closest thing we have to a universal medicine and most people are not taking their dose.

Exercise and Mental Health

This is the one I feel most passionate about, partly because it's the area where exercise most changes lives in ways people don't expect, and partly because it's consistently underestimated.

The evidence for exercise's role in combatting depression is now so strong that it's recommended as a first-line treatment alongside therapy and medication for mild to moderate depression. A major meta-analysis found that exercise was one and a half times more effective at reducing depression and anxiety than medication or psychotherapy alone. And it's free.

Exercise increases serotonin and dopamine, the neurotransmitters most antidepressants target. It reduces cortisol and chronic inflammation, both of which are elevated in depression. It improves sleep quality, which is deeply intertwined with mental health. And it provides something that's harder to quantify but no less real: a reliable, repeatable experience of doing something hard and succeeding at it.

That last one matters. The confidence that comes from showing up to train regularly, from lifting heavier than you did last month, from running further than you thought you could, is transferable. The women I coach who build a consistent exercise habit report changes far beyond their physical appearance. They feel more capable generally. They tolerate discomfort better. They make decisions from a different place.

Making exercise a consistent habit starts with dismantling one belief: that a workout only counts if it's long. It doesn't. Twenty minutes of well-structured resistance training, done consistently three to four times a week, will produce better results than an ambitious hour-long programme you follow for three weeks and then abandon. Consistency beats intensity. Frequency beats duration.

The most common reason women give for not exercising consistently is lack of time. So here is the solution – what I call 'minimum effective dose' workouts, or MEDs for short: three short, sharp, effective sessions per week. Total time commitment: one hour. I want to be clear: will you get optimal results from this? No. I am not the strongest or most muscular person I know. But I do stay in shape year-round while running five businesses and maintaining something that occasionally resembles a social life. MEDs work. For a demonstration, see the videos at this link:

For each workout: 3–4 sets of 10–12 reps, completed as a giant set – circuit-style – with 1–3 minutes of rest between rounds. That's 15–20 minutes. Done.

A few things worth knowing alongside this: you don't need to overdo the protein – most women will get great results aiming for 100g a day. And muscle isn't actually built in the gym. The workout is where you stimulate growth. Recovery is where you grow. Sleep, rest days and adequate food aren't optional extras; they're half the programme.

On resistance training specifically: if you do one thing with your exercise time, make it this. Lifting weights is the single most important training modality for women, particularly as you age. It builds and preserves muscle mass – the primary driver of your resting metabolic rate. It improves insulin sensitivity, bone density and joint health. And the confidence that comes from getting stronger, from lifting heavier than you did last month, transfers into every other area of your life in ways that are difficult to fully explain until you experience them.

Stop Thinking of Exercise as Punishment

The most destructive thing we've done to exercise is turn it into something that women do *to* their bodies rather than *for* them: 'I need to burn off last night's dinner', 'I have to go to the gym because I ate badly this week', 'I deserve a rest day because I've been good'. This framework makes exercise a transaction: you eat something you shouldn't, and you pay for it with movement. And it means exercise is always linked to guilt, restriction and judgement.

When exercise is a punishment, you do the minimum you think you've earned the right to do. You resent it. You avoid it when you're not feeling guilty enough to justify it. You never build the consistent habit that would make it automatic.

When exercise is something you do because you value what it gives you – energy, strength, mental clarity, better sleep, longer life in better health – everything changes. You stop negotiating with yourself. You do it because you want what it gives you, not because you're forcing yourself to. You see it as self-care not punishment.

This reframe is not easy, especially if you've spent years in the punishment mindset. But it's definitely worth working on. Here's how to actually start changing your habits:

- **Track what exercise gives you, not what it burns.** After every session for the next two weeks, write down one thing you got from it. Not the calories burned, but how you felt: more patient with your kids; clearer headed in a difficult meeting; slept better; less anxious. By doing this, you're building evidence that exercise is something that gives you things you want rather than something that makes up for what you ate. Over time, that evidence changes the story.
- **Choose movement you don't hate.** This one sounds obvious but it is consistently ignored. If you dread every session, the problem isn't your discipline, it's the session. You don't have to run if you hate running. You don't have to do classes if you find them excruciatingly boring. The best form of exercise is the one you'll actually do. Start there, and optimise later once the habit exists. Note: if you hate lifting weights, I still would – just do MED workouts (see page 171). The reality is you might not love exercise – not everyone does – but at least do something you don't actively hate.
- **Separate exercise from food entirely.** Stop using workouts to justify meals or to compensate for them. The moment you eat something and think 'I'll need to work that off', exercise becomes punishment by definition. These are two separate inputs into your health, not a transaction. One does not earn or cancel

out the other. Keeping them separate in your mind is one of the most important shifts you can make. Exercise has so many more important and impactful benefits than just burning calories (and it's not even very good at that, as you now know).

- **Notice how much better you show up when you have exercised.** Not in terms of how you look, but in terms of how you are. Are you more patient? More decisive? Less reactive to things that would usually tip you over? Most women I work with report that their relationships, their work and their mood all improve measurably when they're training consistently – and get noticeably worse when they stop. Focus on that immediate benefit from exercise.

The reality is the exercise-as-punishment mindset didn't appear overnight and it won't disappear overnight either. But every time you choose to move because you want what it gives you rather than as a punishment or to earn your next meal, you're rewiring your brain.

Exercise is the closest thing we have to a universal medicine. The dose is movement, the frequency is most days, and the side effects are almost entirely positive.

KEY POINTS

- Fitness is a better predictor of health and longevity than body size. 'Fit and overweight' is healthier than 'lean and sedentary'.
- Exercise reduces the risk of cardiovascular disease, cancer, diabetes, depression, dementia and dozens of other conditions simultaneously. No single drug does this.
- The evidence for exercise in depression is now so strong it's recommended alongside medication and therapy. It's one and a half times more effective in some comparisons.
- The biggest health gains come from moving from nothing to something. The first step is the most powerful.
- Thinking of exercise as punishment produces a resentful relationship with it. Thinking of it as something you do for yourself as self-care produces a sustainable, decades-long habit that you will certainly be grateful for.

Chapter 20

Sleep: The Fat Loss Tool You're Ignoring

I want to ask you something before we go any further: how much sleep did you get last night? And the night before? And what's your honest average across a normal week? For most of the women I work with, the answer is somewhere between five and seven hours, usually fragmented, often disrupted by stress, hormones, a phone on the bedside table or children who have decided that 5:47am is an acceptable time to start the day.

And when I ask these same women what they think is responsible for their hunger, their cravings, their difficulty staying in a calorie deficit, the answers are usually: lack of willpower, emotional eating and not being disciplined enough. Almost nobody says sleep.

They should. Because sleep is one of the most powerful drivers of hunger, cravings, willpower, motivation and discipline, and fixing it – even partially by just improving it – can have a huge impact on fat loss. Of course, life in general is also a lot easier when you have slept well. Poor sleep directly increases hunger hormones, reduces satiety hormones, impairs decision-making and slows recovery from training. Fix your sleep and everything else becomes easier.

What Happens to Your Hunger Hormones When You're Tired

Ghrelin and leptin are the two hormones that act as your body's push and pull on appetite. Ghrelin drives hunger. Leptin suppresses it.

A landmark study published in *Annals of Internal Medicine* in 2004 measured these hormones in men who slept for two nights for four hours compared to two nights for ten hours. The results were stark. After four hours of sleep, ghrelin was up by 28 per cent and leptin was down by 18 per cent. In other words, hunger signals increased and fullness signals reduced – simultaneously. The participants also reported a 24 per cent increase in appetite and showed a clear preference for calorie-dense, high-carbohydrate foods such as sweets, salty snacks and starchy foods. Not increased hunger for broccoli. Increased hunger for exactly the foods that are hardest to eat in moderation when you're trying to manage your intake.

Think about what you actually eat when you're exhausted. It is almost never the chicken and salad you planned. It's toast, biscuits, or whatever is quick and comforting and immediately available. That's not weakness or lack of willpower. That's ghrelin and a depleted prefrontal cortex (the part of your brain responsible for rational decision-making, impulse control and long-term thinking) pointing you directly at the biscuit tin.

What happens in your brain when you are sleep-deprived is not just about willpower running low. The neuroscience is more specific and more sobering than that. A study published in *Nature Communications* used brain imaging to show that after a single night of sleep deprivation, activity in the frontal cortex – the brain region responsible for evaluation, judgement and impulse control – was significantly reduced when participants were shown images of food. At the same time, activity in the amygdala – the brain's emotional response centre – was amplified. The part of your brain that weighs up whether something is a good idea gets quieter. The part that responds to immediate reward gets louder.

The researchers found this shift was associated with a significant increase in desire specifically for high-calorie foods – not food in general, but the highest-calorie options available. A separate study at the University of Chicago went further: participants who were sleep-restricted chose snacks with 50 per cent more calories and twice the fat content compared to when they were well rested – and this was after they had already eaten a meal covering 90 per cent of their daily calorie needs. They were not hungry. They were sleep-deprived. The mechanism appears to involve the endocannabinoid system – the same neural pathway activated by cannabis – which is why the cravings after a bad night of sleep feel remarkably similar to the munchies.

Meta-analyses across multiple studies estimate that experimental sleep deprivation increases daily caloric intake by an average of 385 calories. That is the difference between a deficit and maintenance for many women.

Sleep and Decision Fatigue

Your prefrontal cortex is extraordinarily sensitive to sleep deprivation. After a poor night's sleep, your ability to make good decisions reduces significantly, and the degradation compounds through the day. Every food choice, every workout decision, every moment of resisting a craving draws from a resource that was already depleted before you got out of bed.

This connects directly to what we explored in Chapter 14. The women who tell me they 'just don't have the energy' to stick to their nutrition or get to the gym – they're often not wrong. But the energy problem frequently starts the night before. You can't make good decisions from a cognitive overload. And poor sleep puts you in cognitive overdraft before the day has started.

A 2012 study found that sleep-deprived participants show significantly greater activation in the reward centres of the brain in response to high-calorie food images compared to well-rested participants. The food literally looked more appealing when they were tired. Their brains were working against them. And no amount of motivation or discipline overrides that kind of neurological reward amplification.

Sleep, Cortisol and Fat Storage

Poor sleep raises cortisol. I know we've already spent time on cortisol in Chapter 8, and, as I said there, cortisol doesn't directly block fat loss. But the downstream effects of chronically elevated cortisol matter, and sleep deprivation is one of the most consistent ways to keep cortisol elevated.

Elevated cortisol from poor sleep contributes to water retention (which masks fat loss on the scales), increases appetite particularly for energy-dense foods, reduces motivation to exercise and impairs recovery from training. It creates the worst conditions possible for consistent fat-loss behaviour, day after day.

There's also evidence that sleep deprivation specifically impairs fat oxidation – the process of using fat as fuel. A study in *Annals of Internal Medicine* found that when people were in a calorie deficit but sleeping only 5.5 hours versus 8.5 hours, the composition of what they lost changed significantly. The sleep-deprived group lost 55 per cent less fat and 60 per cent more lean muscle mass than the well-rested group – on the same calorie deficit.

Sleep doesn't just support fat loss. It determines what you actually lose.

How Much Sleep Do You Need?

The research is clear on this even if the wellness industry muddies it with morning routines and biohacking. Most adults need between seven and nine hours of sleep per night. This is not negotiable based on how busy you are. Seven to nine hours is not a luxury for people with uncomplicated lives. It's a biological requirement for basic metabolic and cognitive function.

If you get below six hours consistently, you're operating with measurably impaired cognition, elevated hunger hormones, reduced insulin sensitivity, higher cortisol and worse recovery from exercise. And the insidious thing about sleep deprivation is that you adapt to feeling tired. You stop noticing how impaired you are because it becomes your baseline. You think you're fine on six hours because you no longer remember what functioning properly feels like.

I say this as someone who has gone through phases of terrible sleep. The difference in how I eat, how I train, how I make decisions and, honestly, how I feel about my body when I'm sleeping well versus when I'm not is more dramatic than almost any other variable. It's the part of my routine I protect most fiercely, because everything else runs better when it's right.

Practical Sleep Priorities

I'm not going to give you a 47-step sleep hygiene protocol, because you won't follow it and the complexity isn't necessary. Instead, I'm going to explain the levers with the best evidence and the biggest impact.

Keep a consistent wake time

This is the single most evidence-based sleep intervention, and it's free. Your body's sleep–wake cycle is anchored to your wake time, not your bedtime. If you wake at the same time every day – yes, including weekends – your sleep pressure builds correctly and falling asleep becomes easier. Inconsistent wake times (sleeping in at weekends, which seems logical but is actually damaging) disrupt your circadian rhythm in a way that makes everything harder.

Protect the 90 minutes before bed

Your temperature needs to drop slightly to initiate sleep. Bright light (especially screens), intense exercise, alcohol and heavy meals all interfere with this. You don't need a rigid protocol that's unrealistic and adds stress. You just need a rough wind-down that tells your nervous system the day is ending. This could be reading, taking a shower, going for a walk – anything without a screen.

Address the obvious blockers

For many women, the biggest sleep disruptors are not fixable by a better bedtime routine. They're caffeine consumed after 2pm, alcohol (which fragments sleep architecture even when it seems to help you fall asleep), an environment that's too warm or too bright, kids, a busy life, work and, for perimenopausal women, hot flushes that wake you repeatedly through the night. If it's the last one, that's a conversation with your GP about hormone replacement therapy (HRT), not a sleep hygiene problem.

And on stress: the single biggest thing I hear from women who sleep badly is that they lie awake thinking: racing thoughts, replaying the day, catastrophising tomorrow. If this is you, some version of a brain dump – writing down your thoughts and tasks before bed rather than trying to hold them in your head – consistently outperforms every other intervention I've seen for this specific problem. Get it out of your head and onto paper. Then your brain can stop trying to remember it.

If you feel exhausted and you're trying to do it all, focus on improving your sleep. It's like sharpening that axe before you chop the tree – everything will become easier and more doable.

Sleep deprivation raises ghrelin, lowers leptin, elevates cortisol and amplifies food cravings – and it makes fat loss harder.

KEY POINTS

- Sleep deprivation raises ghrelin by up to 28 per cent and lowers leptin by up to 18 per cent, simultaneously increasing hunger and reducing satiety signals.
- Poor sleep depletes the cognitive resources needed to make good food choices – the fatigue and the cravings are connected, not separate problems.
- Research shows that people in a calorie deficit who are sleep-deprived lose 55 per cent less fat and significantly more muscle than those sleeping adequately. Same deficit. Radically different outcomes.
- Most adults need seven to nine hours' sleep. Below six hours consistently produces measurable impairment in hunger hormones, insulin sensitivity and decision-making.
- A consistent wake time is the single most evidence-based sleep intervention. Anchor your wake time and your sleep will regulate around it.

Chapter 21

The Ultimate Guide to Reducing Hunger: 13 Factors You Haven't Considered

Managing hunger is without a doubt one of the most important aspects of fat loss. When you are in a calorie deficit, you will feel hungry sometimes. That is normal, inevitable and not a bad thing. The goal of this chapter is not to eliminate that hunger, but to give you the tools to keep it manageable.

If you struggle with hunger, you need to look at these 13 factors because what you eat has a huge impact on how much you eat. I'd bet there are more than a few here you're not currently considering.

1. Food Volume

One of the first signals your body uses to register fullness is the physical stretching of your stomach. The stomach has stretch receptors that send a signal to the brain saying, 'We have food, ghrelin can drop.' This happens regardless of the calorie content of what you've eaten.

So, try to maximise the amount of food you can eat per calorie. Choose foods with high water and fibre content. You can eat a vastly larger volume of broccoli than rice for the same number of calories. By filling your plate with vegetables, salads and broth-based soups, you're physically stretching your stomach and triggering that ghrelin drop without the calorie cost. Research on volumetrics – the science of eating more food for fewer calories – consistently shows this reduces total daily calorie intake without increasing hunger.

2. Fibre

Fibre is one of the most underrated tools in fat loss. And in health generally, but let's focus on what it does for hunger.

Fibre slows digestion, adds bulk to meals and, most importantly, increases your body's natural production of GLP-1. Yes, that's the same compound mimicked by weight-loss drugs like Ozempic and Wegovy. High-protein meals stimulate GLP-1 release, which is part of why protein is so effective at managing hunger. Eating slowly is another contributor – it takes around 20 minutes for the gut to signal fullness to the brain, so slowing down your eating gives the hormone time to do its job (see page 90). And finally, fibre also triggers GLP-1 release, which is another reason why vegetables, pulses and wholegrains keep you fuller for longer than processed foods that have had the fibre removed.

Fibre gives you a natural, side-effect-free boost to your satiety hormones. A review in *Nutrition Reviews* found that increasing dietary fibre by 14g per day was associated with a 10 per cent reduction in energy intake and weight loss over time, without any deliberate calorie restriction.

Lentils, beans, oats, whole grains, vegetables and some fruits – especially raspberries – are your friends here. Aim for at least 25–30g of fibre per day. Across a day, that might look like: a bowl of oats at breakfast (4g), an apple as a snack (4g), a large salad at lunch with chickpeas (8g), and vegetables with lentils at dinner (10g). If that sounds like a lot, start by adding one portion of beans or lentils and one extra serving of vegetables per day and build from there.

3. Viscosity

Viscosity means how thick or solid something is. On a practical level, this mostly means: eat your calories, don't drink them.

Liquid calories – like sodas, juices, fancy coffees and smoothies – are far less satiating than solid food. They bypass the chewing process and move through your stomach quickly, which means the stretch receptors barely register them and ghrelin doesn't drop meaningfully. Your brain essentially doesn't count them, and you'll be hungry again faster. Research comparing solid and liquid meals of identical calorie content consistently shows greater satiety and lower subsequent intake from solid food. If you must have a smoothie, make it thick with fibre and protein to increase its staying power.

4. Palatability

Palatability refers to how rewarding and enjoyable a food is. Highly palatable foods are engineered to be exactly that – a perfect combination of sugar, fat and salt that makes them almost impossible to stop eating. Food scientists call this 'hyperpalatability' and it's no accident; it's by design.

The more exposure you have to highly palatable, ultra-processed food, the more your taste receptors adapt to expect that level of stimulation. Fresh fruit starts to taste bland. Plain yoghurt feels boring. You need increasingly intense sugary and salty flavours to feel satisfied. Reducing your exposure to ultra-processed food recalibrates your palate over a few weeks and fresh, whole food starts to taste better.

5. Protein

We covered protein in detail in Chapter 17, but it's worth mentioning again here as protein has a potent satiating effect. It triggers CCK and PYY, suppresses ghrelin and slows gastric emptying. I want to just stress again, though, that protein's impact on hunger is most significant when you're below the recommended intake. Once you're consistently hitting 100 to 140g per day, adding more has diminishing returns. Hit your baseline consistently every day, and this factor largely takes care of itself.

6. Variety Within Meals

Have you ever been completely full after a main course, only to find you suddenly have room for dessert? That's not greed, it's sensory-specific satiety – a well-documented phenomenon where your appetite for one specific food decreases as you eat it, but your appetite for a different food remains.

At a buffet, this effect goes into overdrive. More variety means more eating, even when your stomach is physically full. The strategy to counter this is: keep your main meals simple and consistent with fewer components and less variety within a single sitting. This naturally reduces calorie intake without requiring any deliberate restriction.

Variety is, of course, important to your diet as a whole, but it's worth noting that the research doesn't suggest you need to hit every food group at every meal. What matters is that across the day you're getting a range of vegetables, adequate protein and a reasonable spread of nutrients. If your breakfast is eggs and toast every day, that doesn't matter as long as your overall diet has variety across the week.

7. Snacking

People who snack frequently tend to consume significantly more calories across the day than they realise – not because snacking is inherently bad, but because it's often mindless. When you don't properly register that you've eaten something, it has less impact on your satiety hormones and you end up eating more later anyway.

Constant snacking also means your blood sugar and insulin never fully settle, which keeps you in a state of low-level hunger rather than allowing you to feel genuinely full and then genuinely hungry again. Eating two to four large, satisfying meals spaced at regular intervals throughout the day – rather than grazing or going long stretches without eating and then having a large dinner – and reducing snacking allows your body to complete the hunger–satiety cycle properly, which makes the whole day easier to manage.

8. Meal Timing

Your hunger follows a circadian rhythm. Your body gets used to receiving food at certain times and prepares for it – ghrelin rises in anticipation of your usual mealtimes. This is actually useful: if you have consistent mealtimes, hunger becomes predictable and manageable. If your mealtimes are chaotic, hunger signals are erratic and harder to distinguish from habit-based urges.

Having roughly consistent mealtimes and stopping eating between meals is hard for the first week or two while your rhythm adjusts, but your body adapts. Think of it like getting over jet lag. It's uncomfortable temporarily, but it recalibrates. After that, you stop getting hunger signals at random times and start getting them when food is actually coming.

9. Food Exposure

As we touched on in Chapter 15, willpower is a finite and depleting resource. Research by Roy Baumeister on ego depletion showed that every act of self-regulation draws from the same limited pool. The more decisions you have to make, the more that pool depletes, and the worse your subsequent decisions become. This is decision fatigue, and it's why your resolve tends to be highest in the morning and lowest in the evening.

The solution is not to have more willpower. It's to engineer your environment so you need less of it. A 2013 study tested a simple question: does where you place food affect how much of it you eat? They put apple slices and carrot sticks either on the table directly in front of participants or two metres away. The people who had the food closer to them ate significantly more of it. When they made the food visible – in a clear bowl rather than covered – intake increased further.

It's evident, then, that proximity and visibility drive consumption, regardless of what the food is. Your brain does not distinguish between 'I want that because I'm hungry' and 'I want that because it is directly in front of me'. It just responds to the presence of food by generating desire for it. This works in both directions. If the food in front of you is healthy, you eat more of it. If the food in front of you is a biscuit tin, you eat more of that.

So, put the fruit bowl on the counter. Put the things you want to eat less of in opaque containers on the top shelf. Keep the food you want to eat at eye level in the fridge. Make the healthy choice the easy choice, and make the less helpful choice require effort. Out of sight genuinely does mean out of mind – this is one of the most reliably effective behavioural interventions in the literature.

10. Eating Speed

It takes approximately 20 minutes for the gut hormones GLP-1 and CCK to travel to the brain and register a 'full' signal after food reaches your small intestine. If you eat quickly, you've consumed hundreds of extra calories before that brake pedal even engages.

Studies consistently show that slow eaters consume less and

report greater satisfaction than fast eaters eating the same food. There are some practical tools to help you slow down your eating: drink water with meals, put your fork down between bites and remove distractions (no phone or TV while eating). If you're still hungry after a meal, wait 20 minutes before deciding to eat more to give your biology time to catch up.

11. Energy Balance

If you're in a very large calorie deficit, you'll feel proportionally more hunger. This seems obvious, but it's worth stating: extreme restriction is counterproductive, not just because it's unsustainable but because the hunger it produces makes adherence much harder.

Think of it like pacing a marathon. You want to run at the fastest pace you can maintain for the whole distance, not sprint the first mile and walk the rest. As I've said, a deficit of 10–20 per cent of your maintenance calories is the sweet spot for most people: meaningful enough to produce consistent fat loss, modest enough that hunger doesn't overwhelm you. Too small and progress is demoralisingly slow. Too large and you'll find yourself unable to sustain it. The right deficit is the one you can actually keep.

12. Low-Carb (Worth Understanding Even If You Don't Follow It)

People on low-carbohydrate diets often report lower hunger, and it's worth understanding why because you can then apply those principles without going fully keto.

Low-carb diets tend to be higher in protein and fibre, have greater food volume (because refined grains are replaced with vegetables), reduce palatability by eliminating many ultra-processed foods and limit variety in ways that reduce sensory-specific satiety. These are factors one to six in this list. You can get most of the hunger-management benefit of low-carb simply by increasing your protein, prioritising fibre and reducing ultra-processed carbohydrates – without eliminating carbs entirely.

13. Your Environment

You eat with your eyes more than your stomach and the research on this is genuinely mind-blowing. A now well-replicated study gave participants soup from normal bowls alongside participants whose bowls were secretly and slowly refilling from beneath the table as they ate, so the bowl never appeared to empty. Those eating from the bottomless bowls consumed 73 per cent more soup than those eating from normal ones. That part is somewhat unsurprising, but they consumed 73 per cent more without realising it, without feeling fuller and without any difference in how satisfied they said they felt afterwards. The researchers concluded that people do not monitor how much they have eaten; they look at the bowl and use that as their cue to stop. The bowl was nearly empty, so they felt they had nearly finished. The bowl was still half full, so they kept going.

In practical terms: use smaller plates and bowls. Not as a trick, but as an environmental design choice. Your brain uses visual completion as a stopping signal.

THE ULTIMATE GUIDE TO REDUCING HUNGER

You have more control over your hunger than you think. These 13 factors are not tricks – they're the science of hunger applied practically. Use them.

KEY POINTS

- Food volume and fibre are the two most underused hunger management tools. Both trigger satiety signals without significant calorie cost.
- Eating speed matters: it takes 20 minutes for fullness hormones to reach the brain. Fast eaters consistently consume more.
- Consistent meal timing makes hunger predictable and manageable. Irregular eating keeps hunger signals erratic.
- Engineer your environment so healthy choices require less willpower – willpower is finite and depletes across the day.
- A deficit of 10–20 per cent of maintenance is the sustainable sweet spot for most people. Extreme restriction creates hunger that undermines adherence.

Chapter 22

F*ck Yes or No

Let's now talk about something that might sound a bit unconventional. It's a rule I borrowed from the self-help author Mark Manson. The original article was about dating: if someone isn't a 'f*ck yes', they're a no. It's about making intentional choices, not wasting time and energy on maybes, and going all-in on the things that genuinely matter to you – which requires saying no to everything that doesn't. Manson applied it to relationships. I'm applying it to food. And it's a very useful framework.

Here's the principle applied to food choices: if you want a cocktail, a burger, some ice cream, a slice of cake, something indulgent, it should be a genuine 'f*ck yes'. If it is, you enjoy the hell out of it, fully and without guilt. If it isn't a 'f*ck yes', it's a no. Simple as that.

This is not about deprivation. It's about choosing your indulgences deliberately and savouring them completely. It's about elevating your treats from mindless consumption to genuine pleasure. It's about intention.

Think about how many times you've eaten something you didn't particularly want. You were already full but the dessert arrived. You weren't really hungry but you ordered something anyway because everyone else was. You ate the biscuits in the meeting not because you wanted them but because they were there. You finished the crisps not because you were hungry or even enjoying them, but from habit and inertia.

None of those were 'f*ck yes' moments. They were 'maybes' and 'shoulds' and 'might-as-wells'. And they cost calories, they cost your deficit and – more subtly – they cost you the sense of being in control of your choices.

Every 'Maybe' Has a Cost

Every indulgence that isn't a genuine yes comes with costs beyond just the calories. There's the mental load of eating something you didn't really want and feeling vaguely unsatisfied anyway. There's the guilt that follows – 'I didn't even enjoy that.' And there's the feeling of being slightly out of control, of being led by habit or social pressure rather than your own genuine desires.

Imagine you have a limited budget for something you love – a holiday, a piece of clothing, a restaurant you've wanted to try. Would you spend it on something you felt lukewarm about just because it was on offer? Or because everyone else was buying it? You'd save it for the thing that genuinely excites you. Or at least you should!

Your food budget works in the same way. When you say yes to something that isn't a 'f*ck yes', you're spending your calorie budget on something mediocre. So save your yes for the things that genuinely deserve it.

What About FOMO?

One of the biggest obstacles to this rule is the fear of missing out. We're conditioned to believe that if we don't take every opportunity for a treat, we'll regret it. That somehow the experience is diminished by passing it up.

But what you're actually missing out on by saying yes to every maybe is the genuine satisfaction of the 'f*ck yes' moments. When every social occasion involves eating and drinking because it's there, none of it is particularly special. When you save your 'yes' for the things that actually deserve it, those things become genuinely pleasurable rather than habitually consumed.

And consider what you're also 'missing out on' when you say yes to a maybe: your deficit for that day, your sense of being in control of your choices, the feeling of knowing your yeses were real. Saying no to a maybe isn't missing out. It's making space for a genuine yes later. And saying no to some unwanted food often means saying yes to your goals.

There is something else worth being aware of: eating with other people makes you eat more. Not a little more. Significantly more. A 2019 meta-analysis published in the *American Journal of Clinical Nutrition*, which pooled data across dozens of studies, found that meals eaten with other people were between 29 per cent and 48 per cent larger than meals eaten alone. Not because people were hungrier or because the food was better. Simply because of the social context.

The researchers describe this as the 'social facilitation of eating' – a deeply human behaviour thought to have evolutionary roots in food sharing, but which in a modern environment of calorie abundance becomes a meaningful driver of overconsumption. The effect is strongest when eating with friends and family, particularly at social occasions and with indulgent foods. You almost certainly do this without noticing. Most people, when asked why they ate more at dinner with friends, say the food was good or that they were hungry, not that the presence of others lowered their self-monitoring and extended the meal.

None of this means that you should eat alone or approach a dinner out like a military operation. It means you should go in with your eyes open, eat intentionally and use the 'F*ck Yes or No' framework before you sit down, not after you have had three glasses of wine and the dessert menu is in front of you.

How to Use It

Create a pause before making the decision. Ask yourself honestly: is this a 'f*ck yes'? Not a 'should I?' Not a 'would it be rude to say no?' Not a 'will I regret not having it?' Is this a genuine yes?

Tune in to your body. Are you actually hungry or is something else driving this – boredom, stress, habit, social pressure? If you're already full, the dessert is probably a no. If nothing on the menu is genuinely calling you, it's probably a no.

Think about what your version of this rule looks like across different situations: the dessert menu at the end of a meal out with friends; the office birthday cake; the glass of wine after work because the day was hard. Apply the rule honestly and you'll find that most of those situations fall clearly on one side or the other.

The ones that genuinely feel like a 'yes' are worth having. The others aren't worth the calorie cost or the mental energy.

As an example, alcohol is never a 'f*ck yes' for me. But ice cream is, as long as it's nice ice cream. The ten-year-old choc ice at the back of my parents' freezer is not a f*ck yes. But the gelato in Venice is.

And when you do say yes – when it genuinely is a 'f*ck yes' – lean in completely. Enjoy every bite. Be present. Don't let guilt in. You made a conscious, deliberate choice and you deserve to enjoy it fully. That's not cheating on your diet. That's living intentionally.

I use this framework constantly. It's created a mental balance that feels easily sustainable. I'm never telling myself I can't have something; I'm asking whether I actually want it. Most of the time, when I'm honest, the answer is: not really. And occasionally, the answer is an unambiguous yes. And then I enjoy it completely.

You're not depriving yourself by saying no to a maybe. Saying no often means saying yes to ending the day closer to your long-term goals, but you don't have to say no all the time. You just have to choose your yeses wisely.

KEY POINTS

- If an indulgence isn't a genuine 'yes', it's a 'no'. 'Maybes' are 'nos' in disguise – they cost calories without providing real satisfaction.
- Every 'maybe' indulgence costs more than calories: it costs your sense of control, your deficit and the full enjoyment of future genuine yes moments.
- FOMO drives us towards maybes. But saying no to a maybe is saying yes to your goals and preserving your budget for a genuine yes later.
- When the answer is a genuine 'f*ck yes', enjoy it completely. No guilt. Conscious, intentional pleasure is part of a sustainable approach, not a deviation from it.
- This framework shifts the internal question from 'Can I have this?' (deprivation) to 'Do I actually want this?' (intention).

PART 5

HORMONES, YOUR CYCLE AND WHAT ACTUALLY CHANGES WITH AGE

This is not the section where I encourage you to ignore everything you've just learned and give you a special female diet or tell you to avoid particular exercises at certain times of the month. That is exactly the kind of misinformation we debunked in Part 2. Instead, I'll give you an honest account of the specific ways in which female hormones, the menstrual cycle, menopause and ageing affect fat loss, so you can adapt the tools you've learned so far for the different stages of life.

Chapter 23

The Monthly Sabotage

If you've ever found yourself standing in front of an open fridge at 10pm, three days before your period is due, wondering what happened to your self-control, this chapter is for you.

In my experience coaching women, this is the time of the month when most women give up on their diets. They overeat, skip the gym, experience lower mood, motivation and resilience, and have their worst body image days. But if we want to get consistent results, we can't be giving up for a week every month. We need to find a way through this.

Let me be clear about something important before we go any further: your hormonal fluctuations do not stop fat loss from happening. They make adherence harder. They make the process feel significantly more difficult at certain times of the month. But they do not change the laws of thermodynamics. Telling women anything different sounds empathetic, but it's actually deeply disempowering.

The reason most women struggle around their cycle is because they're trying to stick to a plan while tired, moody, sometimes in pain, experiencing poor body image and lower motivation. They're trying to be logical at a time when logic is genuinely harder to access. I'm 34 at the time of writing and every single month I'm still surprised by the dramatic change in my mood in the days before my period. I really should be used to it by now.

What's Actually Happening

During the luteal phase, the time between ovulation and your period, progesterone rises. This slightly increases your BMR (see page 12). You might burn an extra 100–300 calories a day. Sounds great – a metabolic boost. Except that same rise in progesterone, combined with a drop in oestrogen, also tends to significantly increase your hunger and cravings. Your body is burning a tiny bit more but also demanding a lot more. You also tend to experience reduced motivation to move, which means energy expenditure from movement can actually drop even as BMR rises slightly.

Then there's serotonin – one of the brain's key mood-regulating chemicals, responsible for feelings of calm, emotional stability and well-being. Levels often dip in the luteal phase, which is why you feel more anxious, more irritable and far more likely to reach for highly palatable, energy-dense food – comfort food. The kind that is extremely hard to eat in moderation.

Added to that there's the water retention. Progesterone can cause you to hold on to significant amounts of fluid. You can wake up three pounds heavier overnight while being in a genuine calorie deficit. It's very common to be losing fat and gaining weight simultaneously in the week before your period. If you don't know this is happening, it looks like failure.

When you combine increased hunger, lower mood, reduced motivation and scales that seem to be mocking your efforts, you get the perfect conditions for all-or-nothing thinking: you feel like you've failed, so you might as well eat the whole bag of chocolate. And you're far less rational when you're in this state, which makes it even harder to reason your way out of it.

What Cycle Syncing Gets Wrong

'Cycle syncing' is the idea that you should adapt your training and nutrition to each phase of your cycle. Influencers and 'wellness' experts – and often even women's health specialists – will often tell you to only do yoga during your luteal phase because high-intensity exercise spikes cortisol and stops fat loss, and to eat specific foods for each phase to balance your hormones. It sounds scientific, but it isn't, at least not in the way it's being sold.

A meta-analysis of studies on exercise performance across the menstrual cycle found that while some women might feel slightly less powerful at certain points, there's no consistent, significant difference in fat-loss outcomes or performance that would justify completely restructuring your training every week. For many women, the suggestion to stop training hard during their luteal phase reduces consistency and results. They do less. They move less. Their deficit shrinks. Progress stalls. And it's attributed to their hormones rather than to the reduction in training volume that was encouraged by well-meaning misinformation. When you compound that monthly reduction in volume over months or years, that can really start to negatively impact your progress.

Cycle syncing is a clever way to sell women a complicated solution to a simple problem. You don't need to sync your life to your cycle. You need to listen to your symptoms and adapt based on how you actually feel.

What Helps Instead

Here's what actually makes a difference.

Use your range targets

This is exactly what your range targets were built for. During the follicular phase – the two weeks after your period when energy is usually higher and hunger is more manageable – aim for your Optimal Targets. This is your window of easiest progress. Use it. In the luteal phase or whenever symptoms are worse for you, shift your intention to your Non-Negotiables. You are still moving forward, just at a slower pace for a few days.

What you are trying to avoid is the all-or-nothing response: the hunger hits, you go over your Optimal, you decide the week is ruined and you significantly overeat for five days. That pattern, repeated monthly, is what stalls progress over time. Replacing it with a planned, intentional shift to your Non-Negotiables keeps you moving forward every single week of the month, not just on the ones when you feel good.

The goal during tough week(s) before your period is not perfection. It's usually getting through with momentum or simply not going backwards depending on how severe your symptoms are.

Know your pattern

Most women have a reasonably consistent cycle. If you know you gain three pounds of water in the week before your period, you're no longer alarmed when it happens. Panic causes the all-or-nothing response. Knowledge removes the panic, and removing the panic keeps you consistent.

Plan for the hunger

Your appetite is going to be higher. This is biological. Work with it rather than pretending it isn't happening. Higher-volume, higher-fibre, higher-protein meals during your luteal phase will help you feel more satisfied without derailing your deficit. Eat more of the filling things. Don't try to white-knuckle through the same meals you'd have in week one of your cycle.

Lower the bar on exercise, not on movement

If a full training session isn't happening because you're exhausted or in pain, that's fine. But try to protect your step count and your general activity. Movement is one of the most effective tools for improving mood, reducing cramps and supporting sleep, all of which deteriorate in the luteal phase.

Don't make decisions based on the scales

The week before your period is one of the worst times to evaluate your progress. The scales are up, your mood is low and your hunger is high. Everything looks worse than it is. Make no decisions during this window. Come back to them in week one of your next cycle when you have access to your full rational brain and the water weight has gone.

Make yourself proud

Finally, try to think about how you want to feel the next week, when your mood lifts. Are you going to be proud that you got your head down and kept going or are you going to be annoyed that you overate, skipped your workouts and let your activity drop?

Anecdotally, I often find my mood and motivation are low that week even if I do increase calories, eat a bit more chocolate and let myself skip the gym. So I just continue to do the things I know will make me feel better and my future self will thank me for – eat well, sleep well, get out for a walk, exercise – knowing that feelings fluctuate and we don't always have to respond to them.

You can be losing fat and gaining weight at the same time in the week before your period. Knowing this is half the battle.

KEY POINTS

- Hormonal fluctuations don't stop fat loss. They simply make adherence harder.
- In the luteal phase, your BMR rises slightly but so does your hunger, significantly. Your body is burning a bit more and demanding a lot more.
- You can wake up two to three pounds heavier overnight in the week before your period while being in a genuine calorie deficit. This is water retention, not fat.
- Cycle syncing has no meaningful evidence base for fat-loss outcomes. It often reduces training volume unnecessarily.
- Plan for the hunger, lower the bar on exercise but protect movement, and make no decisions based on the scales during your luteal phase.

Chapter 24

The Menopause Marketing Con

If you're a woman of a certain age, you've probably noticed that the internet has suddenly decided you're broken. According to social media, your hormones are a ticking time bomb, your metabolism has shut down and if you so much as look at a carbohydrate or a treadmill, you'll store fat forever. You're told to avoid cortisol spikes, stop doing HIIT, quit cardio and only do menopause-specific exercise. While, of course, wearing a weighted vest and buying a £150 supplement protocol. Half the suggestions contradict each other. As a result, women are left confused, overwhelmed and worried about doing the wrong thing. I talk to women who feel like this every single day – women who are now genuinely terrified of going through menopause not because of the symptoms themselves, but because of what they've been told it will do to their body and their ability to control it. That fear is completely understandable – and it makes me angry, because most of it has been manufactured. I call this the Menopause Marketing Con.

People have realised that menopausal women are a huge, underserved demographic who are often struggling and looking for answers. And, yet again, where there is struggle, there is money to be made. The people I call the Menopause Manipulators love to tell you that there isn't enough research on women, which conveniently explains why they have no evidence for their claims, and then sell you a cure for the problem they've just convinced you that you have. Some will even diagnose your cortisol levels or your inflammation based on the fact that you occasionally feel tired or bloated. You know, normal human experiences.

Here's the truth: while there's always room for more research, the idea that we 'just don't know' how menopause affects fat loss is an outdated cop-out. We know exactly what's happening.

What Menopause Actually Is

Before we go any further, it's worth grounding this in what menopause actually is, because a lot of confusion comes from the language used around it.

Menopause is not a disease or a failure. It's a normal life stage, defined retrospectively as 12 months without a menstrual period, marking the end of ovarian oestrogen production. Perimenopause is the transition leading up to this point, often lasting several years, where hormone levels fluctuate rather than simply decline. It's these fluctuations that drive many of the symptoms women experience: disrupted sleep, changes in mood, irregular cycles, shifts in body composition . . . the list goes on.

What matters here is that menopause is a process, not an on–off switch, and it does not suddenly rewrite the rules of physiology. Your body is not becoming incapable of responding to food, movement or training; it is adapting to a new hormonal environment. Understanding this distinction is important as once you stop seeing menopause as something that has gone wrong, it's much easier to focus on what actually helps.

The Science versus the Scams

Let's debunk the most common claims I see when it comes to menopause.

Oestrogen

- **The claim:** oestrogen is protective of muscle and, when it drops, you lose muscle.
- **The false conclusion:** you need a special oestrogen-independent muscle-building plan.
- **The reality:** we don't see significant muscle wastage in women who resistance train through menopause. Oestrogen decline does make maintaining muscle slightly harder, but the response is to lift weights and carefully consider recovery, not to buy a special programme.

Carbs

- **The claim:** menopause causes insulin resistance, so you can't handle carbs.
- **The false conclusion:** you need a menopause keto diet.
- **The reality:** the best way to reduce insulin resistance is to stay active, lift weights and maintain a healthy body composition. Carbs are not your enemy during menopause or at any other time.

Cortisol

- **The claim:** cortisol is higher during menopause, and exercise increases cortisol, so you should avoid strenuous exercise.
- **The false conclusion:** do menopause yoga and weighted walks only.
- **The reality:** strenuous exercise increases your stress resilience. HIIT has been consistently shown to have significant health benefits for women at every age, including during and after menopause. Avoiding it because of a misrepresented cortisol argument will actively harm your health.

Perimenopausal and postmenopausal women don't need a completely different approach to exercise and nutrition. They need their programme adapted around their symptoms, not some blanket menopause rule that stops them doing the things that will help them most.

What Does Change

One of the most frustrating physical changes of menopause is the shift in fat storage. As oestrogen declines, fat tends to migrate from the hips and thighs to the abdomen. This is the 'menopause middle' so many women talk about. But the way you lose that fat hasn't changed. You still need a calorie deficit. What has changed is the context. Your sleep might be disrupted by hot flushes. Your mood might be lower. Your stress levels might be higher. And just like during your menstrual cycle, these symptoms then make adherence harder.

The other major change is that muscle mass becomes harder to maintain and more important than ever. Resistance training during and after menopause is not optional if you want to maintain your muscle, metabolic rate, bone density, strength and long-term independence. This is supported by extensive evidence, but it is exactly what the 'avoid strenuous exercise during menopause' crowd is steering you away from.

Don't Settle for Feeling Crap

Many women accept menopause symptoms as their new normal. They settle for feeling okay at best, usually because they've been told that's just what happens when you get older. It doesn't have to be that way.

Symptoms can be significant and debilitating – and I don't want to gloss over that. Things like hot flushes, brain fog, anxiety and joint pain that all seemingly came out of nowhere can have a real impact on your quality of life. If any symptoms are seriously affecting your day-to-day life, please speak to your GP. HRT has had a rehabilitation in recent years, with evidence now showing that for most women under 60, the benefits significantly outweigh the risks. Treatments are better than they've ever been. You don't have to just put up with your symptoms.

And alongside medical support where needed, diet and exercise in the right dose for you remain the most powerful tools available. Not the latest menopause supplement protocol. Not a hormone-reset detox. Not a cortisol-lowering morning routine.

Strength training, adequate protein, an energy deficit for fat loss, sleep and stress management – the same fundamentals applied with a bit more compassion for where you are right now.

You don't need a special menopause version of everything. You need the same fundamentals, applied with awareness of your current symptoms and a bit more self-compassion. What builds muscle and contributes to fat loss pre-menopause is exactly the same during peri- and post-menopause. Your diet and exercise principles have not changed. How you apply them may need adapting.

KEY POINTS

- Menopause is a normal life stage, not a disease. It changes the context of fat loss, not the principles.
- The menopause marketing industry uses real science to reach false conclusions and sell products women don't need.
- Fat tends to redistribute to the abdomen during menopause. The way you lose it remains the same: a calorie deficit.
- Resistance training becomes more important, not less, during and after menopause. The advice to avoid strenuous exercise is harmful.
- If symptoms are significantly affecting your life, speak to your GP about HRT. Treatments are better than ever and the evidence base is much clearer than it once was.

Chapter 25
How to Age Well

We talk about ageing like it's an inevitable and depressing downhill process. We've been conditioned to believe that muscle loss, a slowing metabolism and declining fitness are just part of getting older and there's nothing we can do about it. One of the most common things I hear from women is: 'I'm doing the same things but getting worse results.' In one sense, that's true. But what if a huge part of this and the physical decline we associate with getting older isn't a biological certainty, but a consequence of years of not challenging our muscles, our hearts and our lungs, and our fat-loss behaviours drifting?

In this chapter we'll look at why fat loss genuinely gets harder with age, what is changing in your body, what is within your control and the evidence on how to age well. But first I want to introduce you to someone who completely shatters the 'it's too late' narrative.

Meet Richard Morgan

At 93 years old, Richard Morgan has the aerobic fitness and body fat percentage of a healthy 30- to 40-year-old. He's a four-time indoor rowing world champion and the subject of a fascinating case study published in the *Journal of Applied Physiology*. But here's the interesting part: Richard didn't start exercising until he was 73. Before that, he'd never trained seriously in his life. He wasn't a lifelong athlete coasting on youthful fitness. He was a man in his seventies who decided to change his trajectory.

When researchers looked at Richard, they found something remarkable. His 165-pound frame was around 80 per cent muscle and 15 per cent fat. His heart rate during a maximal fitness test hit 153 beats per minute, one of the highest ever recorded for someone his age. His oxygen uptake, a key measure of cardiovascular health, looked like that of a typical healthy man in his thirties or forties.

His routine isn't some complex, bio-hacked programme. It's simple and consistent: around 40 minutes of rowing a day, mostly easy with some harder work, basic dumbbell sessions and a high-protein diet. Simple basics, repeated consistently. Which, to me, is inspiring as hell.

Richard is living proof that while you cannot stop the years from passing, you can absolutely impact how you experience them. Even if you're starting at 73.

Richard's story forces us to ask an uncomfortable question: if the physical decline we associate with ageing isn't inevitable, how much of it are we actually choosing by default? Let's look at what the evidence says.

What 'Ageing' Is Actually Made of

The majority of people are not like Richard, and we do see significant physical decline with age in most people. But a huge portion of that decline is not inevitable. It's a consequence of moving less.

The medical term for age-related muscle loss is 'sarcopenia'. From around the age of 30, most people lose muscle mass at a rate of 3–8 per cent per decade. After 60, that rate accelerates. This loss of muscle is the primary driver behind the slower metabolism people complain about. Muscle is metabolically active tissue; it burns energy even when you're sitting on the sofa. Less muscle means a lower BMR, easier fat gain and declining metabolic health.

But research shows that much of this 'age-related' muscle loss is actually disuse-related. We stop challenging our muscles consistently. We move less. We settle into more sedentary lives, and our bodies respond by shedding the expensive, energy-hungry muscle tissue they no longer need. 'Use it or lose it' is the most useful way to understand this.

A landmark study published in *Science* in 2021, looking at nearly 6,500 people aged from eight days to 95 years across 29 countries, found something surprising: our metabolism doesn't actually start to meaningfully decline until after the age of 60. And even then, the decline is around 0.7 per cent per year, and it's almost entirely attributable to loss of muscle mass.

So, why does everyone feel like their metabolism tanked in their thirties and forties? It's not physiology. It's lifestyle: more sedentary jobs, more stress, less sleep, more responsibilities, lower energy and less movement. We're burning fewer calories because we've stopped moving as much, not because our biology has fundamentally changed. That is both frustrating and extremely hopeful, because it means you have far more control than you've been told.

Why Muscle Is the Most Important Investment You Can Make

Muscle does so much more than support your metabolism and help you look lean. It is one of the most powerful tools you have for long-term health.

Muscle is the body's largest site of glucose disposal. When you contract your muscles, you activate glucose transporters that pull sugar from the bloodstream directly into muscle cells, often without even needing insulin. This is why regular resistance training has such a powerful protective effect against type 2 diabetes. And why people who exercise tend to maintain their fat loss much better than those who don't: more muscle means better metabolic function at rest and under load.

Muscle also produces myokines, small proteins released into the bloodstream when you exercise. Some act as natural anti-inflammatories. Others support brain health, immune function and bone density. Skeletal muscle is, in the words of researchers who study it, the body's largest endocrine organ. It is not just tissue that moves you. It is actively communicating with the rest of your body every time you use it.

Bone health is another reason this matters, particularly for women. From your thirties onwards, bone mineral density gradually declines. After menopause, this decline accelerates. The consequence is an increased risk of fractures as you get older, particularly of the hip, spine and wrist. Weight-bearing exercise and resistance training are the most evidence-based interventions for maintaining bone density. More evidenced, in fact, than most medications prescribed for this purpose.

What this means for how you train

The most important shift in your thinking should be this: you're not training to lose weight. You're training to build and maintain the body that will carry you through the next several decades in the best possible health.

Fat loss and a good physique are side effects of that goal. They're not the goal itself. When you train to get smaller, you do the minimum you think you need. When you train to get stronger, you push, you progress and the results in your body composition follow naturally.

Richard Morgan didn't start until 73 and became world class. You are not 'too old'. You are not 'too unfit'. You are not 'too far gone'. Start where you are and build from there. The only version of ageing that's truly inevitable is the one where you don't try.

'I'm Doing Everything the Same but I Can't Lose Weight Anymore'

I get messages like this every single day: 'I'm doing everything the same, but now I'm over 40 and I can't lose weight' or 'I used to be able to eat like this and stay lean. Now nothing is working.'

If that's you, you're not imagining it. Something *has* changed. Fat loss genuinely does feel harder for many women as they get older. And you're surrounded by messaging that's ready to explain why: 'It's your age', 'It's perimenopause', 'It's high cortisol', 'It's inflammation', 'It's insulin', 'It's stress', 'It's an inevitable part of ageing'. When you're tired, low in mood or simply fed up and looking for answers, you're far more vulnerable to these messages. And let's be real, it's often nice and comforting to think it's not your fault, that you have no control and there is nothing you can do – so you might as well lean into it.

It's true that it's not your fault, but you can decide to make it your responsibility and change it if you don't like it. So, as usual, I am going to be honest with you about what's actually going on.

Inflammation and insulin: the story gets told backwards

You'll often hear that inflammation or insulin resistance is blocking your fat loss. This gets the causation backwards.

Inflammation is associated with higher levels of body fat, particularly visceral fat around the organs. But it's the fat that's causing the inflammation, not the other way around. Visceral fat is metabolically active tissue that releases inflammatory signals as fat cells become overfull. Losing that fat reduces inflammation. Inflammation isn't the barrier to fat loss; it's often a consequence of excess fat that resolves as you lose it.

The same applies to insulin resistance. Excess body fat, particularly ectopic fat stored in the liver and muscles, is the primary driver of insulin resistance in the general population. Losing fat improves insulin sensitivity. It's not the insulin resistance that's making you gain fat. It's the combination of excess fat and, often, excess calorie intake.

An analogy I like to use to explain this is that thinking that insulin resistance is stopping you losing fat is like thinking that umbrellas cause the rain. Yes, they often appear together and yes, there is a link, but the direction of causation is important. The rain is the primary cause of the umbrella, much like excess fat is the primary cause of insulin resistance. You can't stop the rain by focusing on removing umbrellas. You don't reduce insulin resistance by focusing on insulin. Instead, you focus on reducing body fat.

What's Really Changed

Several things genuinely do change as we age, but almost none of them directly prevent fat loss. Instead, they make it harder to maintain the behaviours that create a calorie deficit.

Sleep quality

Sleep quality tends to deteriorate with age, disrupted further by perimenopause symptoms in many women. I see this constantly with clients. They come to me frustrated, doing everything right on paper – eating well, training consistently – but not seeing the results they expect. And when I ask about sleep, it's almost always the missing piece. They've normalised feeling exhausted because it crept up gradually, and they didn't connect it to the plateau they're experiencing.

We talked about sleep in Chapter 20, but as a reminder: poor sleep increases ghrelin (the hunger hormone) and decreases leptin (the satiety hormone), making hunger harder to manage. It also reduces energy and motivation, making it harder to exercise and easier to make impulsive food choices. What looks like a willpower problem is often just a sleep problem in disguise. The client who can't stop picking in the evenings, who feels out of control around food after 8pm – more often than not, her sleep has been impacted and she hasn't connected the dots as to how much this impacts fat loss.

Energy

As we saw in Chapter 14, low energy makes everything harder. Harder to push yourself while training. Harder to walk enough. Harder to make good food choices. Harder to track accurately. And when everything is harder, small behaviours drift, often without you noticing. The portions get slightly bigger. The tracking gets slightly looser. The steps get slightly fewer. The energy deficit disappears without anything dramatic changing.

Muscle mass

Muscle mass begins to decline from around the age of 30, at roughly 3–8 per cent per decade – if you're not actively working to maintain it. Less muscle means a lower metabolic rate. If you're eating the same amount you ate five years ago but have less muscle mass, you may now be eating at maintenance – meaning you are consuming roughly the same calories as you're burning, so your weight plateaus – or above your deficit without anything else changing.

Life demands

Life generally becomes more demanding as you age: more responsibilities, more stress and less time for yourself. These things affect your capacity to prioritise your health and they affect your sleep, your cortisol response, your energy levels and your food choices.

None of this is your hormones directly blocking fat loss. Poor sleep, high stress, low mood, low energy and under-recovery make identical behaviours feel dramatically harder and yield worse results.

Think about how many times you've gone for a walk and it's

felt easy. Or finished a gym session feeling strong and energised. Now think about times you've done the same walk or the same workout while exhausted and it felt like a completely different experience. The activity didn't change. You did.

This is usually what's actually happening when someone says they're doing everything the same but can't lose weight. The behaviours have drifted in ways that are hard to see because they've happened gradually.

What You Can Do

Everything I've described above might feel overwhelming or even depressing – there are a lot of factors working against us as we age. However, the good news is that every single one responds to the right behaviours. This is where your power lies.

Protect your sleep

This isn't optional. Sleep deprivation undermines fat loss in multiple ways: it increases hunger hormones, reduces satiety hormones, impairs recovery from training and makes every good decision harder. If your sleep is consistently poor and you're struggling with fat loss, addressing sleep is likely the most impactful single change you can make.

Build and maintain muscle

This is the most powerful long-term strategy for managing your metabolic rate as you age, despite the myth that lifting weights will make women 'bulky'. Resistance training two to three times per week, with a focus on adequate protein (roughly 1.6–2.2g per kilogram of body weight daily – see page 147 for more on this) and progressive overload – gradually increasing the weight or difficulty of your training over time rather than doing the same thing every session – is non-negotiable for women over 35 who want to maintain their body composition. It is also the most underused tool in the female fat-loss toolkit.

The short version: progressive resistance training builds a leaner, stronger body, not a bulky one. It is very hard for women to build muscle, and you certainly won't build it by accident.

Be honest about what 'the same' actually means

'I'm doing the same things as before' is worth scrutinising. Are your portions actually the same? Is your step count actually the same? Is your training intensity actually the same? Often they aren't, not because you're dishonest, but because these things drift slowly over time and we don't notice.

Adjust for where you are now, not where you were

If you have less time to exercise, your programming needs to be smarter. If you're sleeping badly, your hunger will be higher. If your stress is chronically elevated, your capacity for consistency might be lower and you might need to make choices easier by automating them. The programme that worked for you five years ago may need to be recalibrated for your current reality. And it's worth remembering: Richard Morgan didn't start until he was 73. It's never too late!

It's not your hormones directly blocking fat loss. It's the downstream effects of real-life changes making adherence harder. Those things are all addressable.

KEY POINTS

- Sarcopenia, age-related muscle loss, is largely disuse-related, not biologically inevitable. Use it or lose it.
- Muscle is metabolically active, produces health-protective myokines, supports glucose disposal and maintains bone density. It is your most important long-term health investment.
- Train to get stronger and healthier. The body composition follows. That shift in mindset makes all the difference.
- Fat loss does become harder with age, but almost never for the direct hormonal reasons you're told. It's the downstream effects on sleep, muscle mass, energy and adherence that make the difference.
- Explanations that remove your agency – such as, 'It's your hormones, there's nothing you can do' – may feel validating but they actively prevent you from making changes.
- Declining muscle mass is the primary driver of a slower metabolism with age. Resistance training is the solution.
- 'Doing the same things' often isn't quite true. Behaviours drift gradually and invisibly. An honest reassessment is usually more useful than a new protocol.

PART 6

MAKING IT LAST

Losing fat is the part most people focus on, but keeping it off is the part that actually matters. It's the harder part, and the part that most programmes completely ignore. But not this approach and not this time.

Part 6 is about making everything you have built in this book last – not just for six weeks or six months, but for the rest of your life. Maintenance is the whole point. Otherwise it ends up just being another yo-yo dieting attempt. In the chapters to come, I'll show you how to transition out of a deficit, why the majority of people regain weight, what the evidence says about the people who don't and the mindset tool you need to safeguard maintenance for life.

Chapter 26

Why Maintenance Matters

Most people have lost fat before. I'd bet you have. Unfortunately, most people regain the weight they lose. Statistics show that as many as 95 per cent of diets 'fail' – in other words, people regain the weight they lost, and often more. These statistics are frequently used as arguments against dieting altogether. Why would you do something with such a high failure rate? Diets clearly don't work.

A better approach – if you actually want results – is to stop listening to people telling you that you're a victim, that you're incapable of change and that most diets fail. Instead, start asking: why do diets usually fail, and what can I do differently?

A key reason is that most diets are unrealistic and over-restrictive. Diets that exclude major food groups, drastically cut calories and force you to put your life on hold are unlikely to produce long-term results. Unsurprisingly, you end up resenting the process, which makes it a short-term solution by definition.

The other reason is that there's almost no emphasis on what happens after the diet ends. I would argue that the maintenance phase is more important than the dieting phase itself. I want to spend some time on this, because most people treat maintenance as though it's simply the absence of a diet – as though you've crossed a finish line and now you're done. This is why most people regain the weight.

Why Maintenance Matters More than the Loss

Maintaining fat loss is one of the most powerful things you can do for your long-term health. Not losing weight, but maintaining the loss. The two are different, and the health benefits accumulate over years of maintenance in ways that a single successful diet never produces on its own.

Here's what the research shows. Sustained weight loss – not temporary loss, but loss maintained over years – significantly reduces the risk of type 2 diabetes. The Diabetes Prevention Program, one of the largest and most robust lifestyle intervention trials ever conducted, found that participants who lost 5–7 per cent of their body weight and maintained that loss over time reduced their risk of developing type 2 diabetes by 58 per cent. That's more than double the benefit of the best medication trialled in the same study. And the key word here is 'maintained'. The protective effect came from keeping the weight off, not just from losing it.

Maintained fat loss also substantially reduces cardiovascular risk. Sustained reductions in body weight lower blood pressure, improve cholesterol profiles, reduce triglycerides and decrease the chronic low-grade inflammation that drives arterial disease. A post-hoc analysis of the Look AHEAD trial, published in *The Lancet Diabetes and Endocrinology* in 2016, found that participants who achieved and sustained significant weight loss showed meaningful reductions in cardiovascular risk that those who regained weight did not. The protective effect came specifically from keeping the weight off, not just from losing it in the first place. The body recovers, but it needs time at the lower weight to do so – and that time is what maintenance provides.

For women specifically, maintaining a healthy body weight is strongly protective against several hormone-sensitive cancers, including breast cancer, endometrial cancer and ovarian cancer. Excess body fat actively produces oestrogen – it doesn't just sit there passively – and elevated oestrogen can drive the growth of certain hormone-sensitive tumours. Research from the Women's Health Initiative – one of the largest studies of women's health ever conducted – found that postmenopausal women who lost 5 per cent or more of their body weight had a significantly lower risk of developing breast cancer compared to those whose weight stayed stable.

Joint health is another area where weight loss maintenance compounds in the right direction. Each kilogram of body weight exerts roughly 4kg of force on the knee joint during walking. Losing 10kg and maintaining that loss reduces the load on each knee by approximately 40kg with every step you take. Over the course of a day, a week, a decade, that difference in cumulative joint stress is enormous. It's the difference between developing osteoarthritis in your fifties or your seventies. Between needing a knee replacement and not.

And then there's metabolic health broadly. Maintaining fat loss over years improves insulin sensitivity, reduces visceral fat and keeps fasting glucose, fasting insulin and inflammatory markers in healthier ranges. These are not numbers that appear on the scales. They're not visible. But they are so much more important: they provide the biological underpinning of how you feel every day and how long you remain healthy and independent. Maintenance is active, ongoing investment in all of those outcomes.

The Hidden Cost of Weight Cycling

There is a specific reason I am so committed to helping people maintain their results rather than simply lose weight, and it goes beyond the obvious. It's the damage that repeated weight cycling – losing and regaining, losing and regaining – does to the body over time.

Weight cycling, often called yo-yo dieting, is not a neutral process. It's not simply that you end up back where you started. Each cycle tends to make the next one harder, and the health consequences accumulate in ways that most people are completely unaware of.

Research on weight cycling is concerning. Studies suggest that repeated cycles of losing and regaining weight may be associated with higher cardiovascular risk and mortality, independent of final body weight, though findings across the literature are not entirely consistent. What the evidence does clearly support is that sustained fat loss produces better long-term health outcomes than repeated short-term losses followed by regain.

Part of this is cardiovascular. Each weight loss and regain cycle appears to increase arterial stiffness and impair endothelial function – the flexibility and responsiveness of the blood vessel walls that are fundamental to cardiovascular health. Part of it is metabolic: repeated cycles of restriction and refeeding alter insulin sensitivity and fat distribution in ways that make subsequent fat loss harder and fat regain faster. And part of it is compositional: when you lose weight rapidly and regain it, you typically regain a higher proportion of fat relative to muscle than you lost, meaning your body composition deteriorates with each cycle, even if your scale weight returns to the same point.

I'm not telling you this to add to your anxiety or to make you feel like past attempts have permanently damaged you. That is the last thing I want. The research also shows that the body is remarkably resilient, and that breaking the cycle – committing to a sustainable loss and maintaining it – reverses much of this damage over time. But it does underline why I place so much emphasis on maintenance. Losing weight and regaining it, losing it and regaining it, over and over again, is not a neutral process that simply resets back to zero. It has a cost. Maintaining the loss breaks that cycle permanently. That's worth understanding clearly.

The Long Game

The biggest mistake people make when they reach their goal weight is treating maintenance as a state of passive continuation. It is not. Maintenance is an active practice, especially given the environment we live in where the preset, the average, the norm is being overweight and inactive. You will always have to apply some effort to actively work against that. Many people insinuate that once you nail this there will become a point where it's easy, where all your habits are automatic, but I am going to be real with you: I have been in shape for over a decade and it's not easy. And I am someone who likes exercise. This isn't to be discouraging, it's to be realistic and to make sure you don't feel like a failure for not suddenly finding it easy. You will still have cravings, you will still have urges, there will still be days, weeks and maybe even months where your motivation for the gym is low. I feel all of this too. That means we need a plan not just to lose fat, but to maintain it.

My whole coaching approach, and more broadly the impact I want to have, is to help people achieve long-term results. To put an end to the constant yo-yo dieting that has sadly become such a huge part of so many women's lives. There are two key elements when it comes to this: the practical side and the mindset side, which we'll cover in the following two chapters.

Everyone wants to know how much they can lose in six weeks. The question that actually matters is how much they'll still have kept off in six months, or six years. The answer to that question is determined almost entirely by what happens after the fat-loss phase ends.

You've done the hard part. You've learned how your body works, what hunger really is, how to manage difficult days, how to build habits and how to think about food differently. That knowledge doesn't expire. Use it for the rest of your life.

You have probably lost weight before. That isn't the impressive part. The impressive part is keeping it off. And that requires a plan.

KEY POINTS

- Most diets fail not because fat loss is impossible but because there's no plan for what happens after – yet the maintenance phase is more important than the fat-loss phase.
- Sustained fat loss – not just losing weight, but keeping it off – reduces risk of type 2 diabetes by up to 58 per cent, significantly lowers cardiovascular risk and is protective against hormone-sensitive cancers.
- Weight cycling has its own independent health costs, including increased cardiovascular risk and worsening body composition with each cycle. Breaking the cycle with genuine maintenance reverses this.

Chapter 27

What People Who Successfully Maintain Actually Do

We don't have to guess at what practical steps maintenance requires. We have good data on it, largely from a long-running research initiative called the National Weight Control Registry (NWCR) – the largest ongoing study of successful long-term weight loss maintainers in the world. To be included in the registry, participants must have lost at least 13.6kg and kept it off for at least a year. The average participant has lost around 30kg and maintained that loss for over five years. These are genuinely successful maintainers, and the researchers have been studying what they have in common since 1994.

The findings are both reassuring and instructive – reassuring because there's no magic, and instructive because the patterns are consistent and replicable. Let's have a look at the most common behaviours.

Eat breakfast

Approximately 78 per cent of registry participants eat breakfast every day. This isn't because breakfast is metabolically special – the research on breakfast timing and metabolism is more nuanced than the headlines suggest – but because consistent breakfast eating tends to anchor the rest of the day's structure. People who skip breakfast are more likely to make impulsive food choices later. It's the consistency that matters, not the breakfast itself, which links very nicely to the 3:1 method.

Stick to a familiar rotation of meals

Registry participants also consistently report eating a relatively low variety of foods. This connects directly back to what we covered in Chapter 21 – variety within meals drives greater calorie intake. Successful maintainers tend to eat a familiar rotation of meals, particularly during the week, with more flexibility at weekends and social occasions. That's essentially the 3:1 method in practice.

The good news is that the 3:1 method isn't just a fat-loss tool. It's one of the most effective frameworks for long-term maintenance precisely because it's a way of eating, not a diet. And it works long term. At maintenance, you simply adjust the flexibility window slightly – a little more at dinner, perhaps a slightly larger snack. The structure of the day stays the same. The habit is already built. The decision-making overhead is already eliminated. Moving from a fat-loss phase to maintenance using this method is a small calibration, not a complete overhaul. That continuity is exactly what most maintenance approaches are missing.

It's often promoted that you should gradually increase calories in small increments after a deficit. There's no need to do this. You can go straight to your estimated maintenance calories. You don't need to slowly edge them up. You'll simply be in a deficit for longer than necessary if you do. With my own clients, I'll usually err slightly on the side of caution and bring calories up to just below their predicted maintenance to allow for inaccuracies, then increase if needed.

If you've been tracking calories during fat loss, keep tracking for at least six weeks at maintenance. You need to understand what maintaining actually looks and feels like before you remove the scaffolding.

Self-monitor

Around 75 per cent of registry participants weigh themselves at least once a week. This is one of the most reliably replicated findings in maintenance research. Regular self-monitoring – tracking the data, noticing trends, catching creep early – is strongly associated with successful long-term maintenance. The people who stop monitoring are the people who most often regain. Not because the monitoring causes the maintenance, but because it reflects the level of ongoing attention that maintenance requires.

After moving to maintenance, I therefore recommend continuing to weigh yourself daily and take the lowest weight of the week for at least six weeks, and using performance markers to assess your body composition thereafter, whether that is in the gym, progress photos, how your clothes fit, your energy or something else – like being able to squat your own body weight or do at least three press-ups. My top tip would be to consider them all as they all matter and tell you whether you're maintaining muscle in a way the scales can't.

Exercise

Around 62 per cent of the participants watch fewer than ten hours of television per week, and 90 per cent exercise for approximately one hour per day on average. The exercise finding is important because the type of exercise reported by most registry members is not extreme training or spending hours in the gym, but walking. Consistent, moderate daily movement is what characterises successful maintainers, not athletic intensity. This aligns with everything we've covered already about the importance of NEAT (page 12) and the sustainability of habits over time (page 135).

For maintenance, you need to keep maintaining your activity. Specifically, continue resistance training two to three times per week, keep your daily step count consistent and resist the temptation to drop exercise now that you've 'finished'. The people who successfully maintain are the ones who continue to exercise consistently. When it comes to muscle, it's as simple as this: use it or lose it.

Protect your sleep

Maintenance requires the same sleep focus as fat loss: aim for seven to nine hours, protect your sleep environment and treat chronic poor sleep as the problem it is rather than a badge of how busy you are.

Keep stress in check

Chronic high stress increases appetite and food intake, and thus drives fat storage, particularly around the abdomen. The stress management tools in Chapter 8 are not just for fat loss; they are for maintaining your results. If your stress levels rise significantly, your maintenance will feel harder and it's very common to regain the weight. Note: not because stress alone causes weight gain, but because of the impact on your behaviours.

What to Expect When You Move to Maintenance

There are specific, predictable things that happen when you bring your calories up to maintenance. Knowing about them in advance means you won't panic and do something counterproductive.

Weight gain

You will gain weight when you bring your calories up to maintenance – and this is not body fat. It's glycogen (your carbohydrate stores refilling), it's water (glycogen requires water to store, roughly 3g per gram) and it's food volume – you're simply eating more. Many people don't expect this weight gain, assume they're doing something wrong and immediately drop their calories again. It's important you don't do this.

Dropping your calories again the moment you see a small gain triggers the same cycle that caused the original problem. Your body needs time to adapt to the higher intake. If you restrict again every time there is a little increase on the scales, you end up in a vicious cycle. Trust the process and give your body at least four to six weeks at maintenance before making any further adjustments.

Note: it is very normal for your maintenance weight to be higher than the weight you finish dieting on – give yourself a buffer of at least a few pounds given that weight fluctuations will still happen, which brings us on to my next point.

Weight fluctuations

Your weight will always fluctuate, sometimes even more than it did during active fat loss, simply because you have more calories and therefore more variation in food volume and water retention.

This is not failure. Average your weight across the week, compare week on week, and remember the rule from Chapter 4: short-term fluctuations are not body composition changes. It's so important to remember this as women get so hung up on the scales: you have to accept that your weight will fluctuate.

A need for structure

Most people regain weight during their maintenance phase because they lose all structure the moment the 'diet' ends. They stop planning meals, stop prepping, stop tracking, stop thinking about protein and fibre. The likelihood is – especially for women who have fewer calories to play with and therefore a smaller absolute deficit – that your maintenance diet is going to look very similar to your fat-loss diet. Just with a little more food.

This third point deserves more than a paragraph, because it's where almost everyone goes wrong and yet it's the most preventable failure in the whole process.

Think about what actually changed during your fat-loss phase. You started planning meals. You got deliberate about protein. You started thinking about food volume. You used the structured approach of the 3:1 method. You built a rough routine around your eating. You got better at estimating portion sizes. You became more aware of the relationship between what you eat and how you feel. All of that was the work. And all of that needs to continue at maintenance – just calibrated to a slightly higher calorie target.

Your maintenance diet looking similar to your fat-loss diet isn't a punishment. It isn't a sentence of perpetual restriction. It's simply the reality that the habits which produced the result are the habits that maintain it – with slightly more food, and considerably more flexibility, but the same underlying structure. Once those habits have genuinely automated – and for most people that takes one to two years – the active effort required reduces significantly. You're not tracking every day forever. You're building a new normal that eventually requires very little conscious effort to sustain.

Weight regain

It is very normal and human for you to start to drift towards regaining weight. It happens to everyone. The difference is that you are going to course-correct quickly. If your weight starts trending upwards over four to six weeks of maintenance, that is your early warning signal. Do not ignore it, but do not panic. Simply tighten your structure and do a bit of an audit. Spend a week or two being more mindful of your intake and output and make sure you're still ticking the boxes. Small adjustments made early are far easier than a full fat-loss phase repeated from scratch. This is exactly why it's important to check in with yourself, or your coach if you have one, and monitor progress. That way you catch the drift in behaviours early before it has time to have much impact.

People who regain weight rapidly after a diet almost universally describe the same pattern: they stopped all monitoring, stopped planning, stopped thinking about it, and slowly drifted back to the eating habits that produced the original weight gain in the first place. Of course they regained – they removed every system that was producing a different outcome.

Research consistently bears this out. A 2014 study found that the single strongest predictor of weight regain at one year was the degree to which participants had reduced their self-monitoring behaviours – tracking, weighing, planning – compared to their fat-loss phase. Not how much they'd lost. Not how fast they'd lost it. How much attention they stopped paying.

The practical takeaway from the NWCR data is this: people who maintain their weight long-term tend to eat regularly (not erratically), weigh themselves frequently (at least weekly), exercise consistently, watch less television and have a plan they can return to quickly after disruption. None of these are surprising. But the research confirms that they are the things that actually matter, not the specific diet approach used. So, when it comes to maintaining your results, the actions and behaviours that got you there will keep you there – usually the biggest shift is you get to eat a little more.

There is no end point. Health and fitness are not things you ever finish. You are never permanently done taking care of your body.

KEY POINTS

- Research from the National Weight Control Registry shows that successful long-term maintainers consistently weigh themselves, eat breakfast, do daily moderate exercise and keep a familiar food routine – simple, sustainable habits, not extreme ones.
- There's no need to slowly increase your calories over weeks – this will just prolong the time you are spending in a deficit unnecessarily. Go straight to your estimated maintenance calories and adjust from there.
- Your maintenance diet will look very similar to your fat-loss diet. The habits that produced the result are the habits that maintain it – slightly more food, same underlying structure.

Chapter 28

F*ck Average: The Maintenance Mindset

Health and fitness are not things you ever finish. Read that again. You are never permanently 'done' taking care of your body. Just like learning, self-development, relationships or parenting, you have to continue working on this. You don't reach a point where it maintains itself, much like you can't trim your hedge into the perfect shape and then put the shears away forever. It will only stay that way with consistent, ongoing trimming. It needs care and maintenance. So do you.

The mistake most people make is treating diet and exercise like they have an end date. Like something to endure until they can stop. But it doesn't end, which means the approach needs to be one you can sustain indefinitely. If you've been white-knuckling a diet you hate for 12 weeks, the maintenance phase is going to be very short.

The goal isn't to be finished. It's to build a way of living – eating, exercising, sleeping, moving – that you can repeat day after day without burning out. One that you actually enjoy. One that supports your energy, your health and the life you want. When you stop chasing an end point and start embracing the daily practice, and appreciating the immediate reward of how you feel rather than waiting for a future destination, progress becomes both inevitable and sustainable. That's the clicking point. Embracing that mindset is how you get long-term results.

A New Identity

We looked at the findings from the NWCR in the previous chapter, but what's also notable is what long-term maintainers report about how maintenance *feels*. After two to five years, the majority report that maintenance feels easier than the active fat loss phase did. The habits have automated, the food environment has been restructured and their identity has shifted – they no longer think of themselves as someone who lost weight and is trying to keep it off. They simply live this way.

The women I have worked with who maintain their results long term say the same: they treat maintenance as a permanent relationship with their health and realise there is no end point to looking after yourself and your body. And over time, it stops feeling like a framework or a diet at all. It just becomes how they live and part of who they are. That identity shift is your goal. And it takes time, which is why the early years of maintenance require the most deliberate support.

The most durable behaviour change happens at the level of identity, not outcome. Every action you take is a vote for the kind of person you believe yourself to be. When you consistently eat well, you're not just eating well that day, you're casting a vote for the identity of someone who eats well. When you exercise consistently, you're not just completing a workout, you're reinforcing the belief that you're someone who moves their body. Over time, enough votes accumulate that the identity becomes settled. And a settled identity is far more durable than motivation or willpower.

This is why the early years of maintenance are the most important and the most fragile. That identity is still forming. The habits are automated in principle but not yet deeply ingrained. The old environment and old social dynamics can easily pull you back into old patterns. This is when structure, accountability and support matter most – not because you don't trust yourself, but because you're still building the new self you're trying to become.

I want to tell you about a mentality that will help you build this new identity and change how you approach maintenance, how you make decisions, what standards you hold yourself to, how you respond when things are hard and ultimately how you get the most out of life. I call it 'f*ck average'. And before you think this is just motivational fluff, it isn't – well, maybe it is a bit, but it works.

F*ck Average

The premise is simple: average is what happens when you stop making active choices and just let the current take you. F*ck average is the decision to be different. Not because you want to be better than other people, or because you think you're special, or because you want to spend your life grinding relentlessly without joy. But because you respect yourself enough to want more. Because you know that the version of your life on the other side of consistent intentional effort is dramatically better than the one you get by going with the flow. And because life is genuinely, finitely short – and you want a good story to tell with minimal regret when you look back on it.

What you miss when you settle for average

Average isn't a comfortable resting place. It looks like one from the outside: everyone's doing it, little is required of you, there's no pressure, you don't stand out and no one judges or questions your choices. But average produces its own very specific discomforts: the low energy that makes getting through the day feel like wading through mud; the quiet frustration of knowing you could be doing more; the cycle of starting and stopping and starting again; the feeling of living slightly below your own potential, indefinitely; the subtle voice in the back of your head telling you that you're not fulfilling your potential, you're not making the most out of life.

The f*ck average life is harder in some ways. Of course it is. It's harder to get up and go to the gym than to stay in bed. It's harder to say no to the third slice of pizza than to eat it. It's harder to not give in to peer pressure when drinking doesn't align with your goals. It's harder to work on your goals when everyone around you has clocked off for the day. But in some ways it's easier. There's a satisfaction you feel when you know you've done your best. You get to go to bed contented and there is a peace in that.

Nothing truly rewarding happens without hard work. Not a healthy body, not a strong relationship, not a successful business, not an impressive skill, not a life you're proud of. The hard things and the good things are the same things. There is nothing I have that I am truly proud of that I haven't worked hard for. The value is often in the work you're avoiding. When something feels hard, that's the signal that you're doing something worth doing; it's the evidence that you're pushing yourself.

If you don't want average results, you can't put in average effort. That's the reality.

If you want to be healthy, you can't be normal

Here's a truth about modern life: the default in the UK is unhealthy, under-energised and often unfulfilling for many people. Being 'average' means being overweight, inactive, chronically stressed and either yo-yo dieting or having given up on the idea of feeling good in your body. It means drinking too much on weekends, eating ultra-processed food as the staple of your diet and lulling yourself into a false sense of security because 'it's the norm'.

We've normalised poor sleep ('everyone's tired'). We've normalised chronic stress ('that's just life'). We've normalised diets built around ultra-processed food ('everything in moderation'). We've dressed it up as balance and self-care, when often it's just comfortable avoidance.

We are wired to follow social norms. From early childhood, we learn through observation and imitation – it's one of the most fundamental human learning mechanisms. We watch what others do, often without conscious awareness, and follow suit. Because everyone else is doing it, we let ourselves off the hook. It feels safe. It feels acceptable. It feels like it can't possibly be a problem if it's this widespread.

But the default option in our current environment is almost always the unhealthy one: processed, calorie-dense, convenient food is everywhere, cheap and aggressively marketed; sedentary behaviour is the path of least resistance; alcohol is woven into nearly every social occasion. None of this is accidental – it's the result of decades of commercial decisions that prioritise profit over public health.

Research on social norms and eating behaviour is clear: we eat more in groups, we eat what the people around us eat and we unconsciously adjust our intake to match the people we're with. If your social environment normalises large portions, frequent treats and sedentary evenings, that becomes your baseline too because you're human and responsive to your environment.

There's a concept in behavioural science sometimes referred to as the 'friend of a friend' effect. Large social network studies have shown that behaviours like weight gain, smoking and even happiness spread through social groups. If a friend becomes obese, your likelihood of becoming obese increases. If a friend of a friend becomes obese, your risk still increases. Even three degrees of separation can have an influence. Not because anyone is copying deliberately or because obesity is contagious, but because norms quietly shift.

Importantly, researchers propose that this is not simply about shared environments, but about shifting social norms. As perceptions of what is a 'normal' body size and eating behaviour change within a network, individual behaviour adjusts accordingly. In other words, we do not just mirror the people beside us; we absorb the standards of the social world we are embedded in.

When the people around you change what they see as normal, your perception of normal changes too. Portion sizes drift. Activity levels drift. Attitudes towards food drift. The powerful part of this research isn't that you're doomed by your circle – it's that environments shape outcomes more than most of us realise. And that the reason for this is that we don't question social norms, we just go with the flow. The answer isn't to hope that your environment will just magically change or wait for government policy to fix it for you. That is never going to happen – not fast enough for any of us alive today. The answer is to open your eyes and take responsibility yourself.

Your environment has more power than you think

I've spent time in Cape Town, Mexico and Sydney and found it remarkably easy to exercise daily, eat well and stay active. It required almost no willpower because that was simply the default. People were walking and cycling everywhere, eating fresh food and exercising outdoors. The environment made healthy choices the path of least resistance.

The UK in January is not the same: grey skies, rain, comfort food culture, pubs on every corner, offices stocked with biscuits, commutes that require no physical activity – and more rain. The environment constantly nudges you in the opposite direction. If you've ever thought 'it feels genuinely hard to get in shape', you're absolutely right. It is harder, because everything around you is pushing back.

But you can change your environment, even if you can't move to a sunnier climate. I'm not talking about dramatic overhauls, but small, deliberate changes to the immediate environment that shift what the path of least resistance actually is:

- Meet friends for walks instead of coffee and cake.
- Join a run club or gym class where the social norm is exercise.
- Organise active social events.
- Get a walking pad for online meetings.

- Remove the biscuit tin from the kitchen counter and replace it with a fruit bowl.
- Sit near the people at work who eat well rather than next to the person who always has chocolates.
- Surround yourself with people for whom healthy behaviour is the norm and is a priority.

That last one is probably the most powerful of all – if your close friends are active and eat well, it becomes far easier to do the same without effort or willpower. You're not swimming against the current anymore, you can go with the flow. And I am not suggesting you ditch all your mates because they aren't HYROX athletes. You can be the change. You can create the social norms. You can be the positive influence.

If you don't want to be average and you want to stay in maintenance, you need to start living your life intentionally – in line with your values and what is actually most important to you. Rejecting the norm starts when you stop settling for what everyone else is doing and start asking what actually serves you.

That might sound judgemental. It isn't. I genuinely don't care how other people choose to live their lives – it's completely their choice and none of my business. The problem is that so many people aren't consciously choosing. They're just floating. And floating in the current direction takes you somewhere most people don't actually want to end up.

What real balance looks like

Real balance – and I mean genuine balance, not the version used to justify daily treats and skipped workouts – is a life where you feel energised, strong and at home in your body. A life where you're not constantly battling yourself. Where healthy choices are the default rather than the exception. Where you feel genuinely well most of the time.

That life doesn't require perfection. It doesn't require being the fittest person in every room or eating impeccably at every meal. It requires building habits and an environment where healthy is simply how you tend to live – and unhealthy is the occasional conscious choice that you enjoy fully (the 'f*ck yes' from Chapter 22) rather than the constant background hum of your existence.

Getting there requires being different. It requires going against some social currents. It requires the courage to decline things, to change how you spend time, to choose differently from the people around you on some occasions. That's genuinely uncomfortable sometimes, but it gets easier. And the life on the other side of that discomfort is worth it.

If you don't want average outcomes, you cannot behave like the average person. And if you want an extraordinary life, it's likely going to require extraordinary effort. This is true for all areas of life, not just fat-loss maintenance. We are often told well-meaning things like 'don't work too hard' or 'set strong boundaries', but most things in life that are worth having do require hard work. And those well-meaning messages are often costing you your potential. There is nothing wrong with a little hard work. It doesn't have to be 'toxic'.

The Five Principles of F*ck Average

Over the years, I've distilled the f*ck average mentality into five core principles. These aren't 'rules' to follow perfectly. They're orientations – the direction you're pointing in, even on the days when execution is imperfect. In fact, as you should know by this point, *especially* on those days!

1. Do what most people avoid

Take risks. Start the thing. Exercise daily. Fuel yourself properly. Say no to the things that don't give you energy or align with your goals. Read, learn, grow. Wake up early and move. Show up even when it's inconvenient. Success is consistently found by doing the opposite of what most people do – and the beautiful thing is that because most people avoid so much, the bar for standing out is genuinely low. You don't have to be extraordinary. You just have to be consistent.

2. Imperfect action beats perfect inaction every single time

Showing up daily and doing your best matters infinitely more than showing up perfectly on the rare occasions when conditions are ideal. Perfectionism is just an excuse to quit when you can't be perfect – and you will never be perfect, so perfectionism is essentially a permanent excuse to give up. Do what you can in the situation you're in. The ten-minute workout is better than no workout. The imperfect meal is better than the full-on biscuit binge. The imperfect attempt is better than the paralysed waiting.

3. Hold high personal standards

Your standards decide your results. Every time you bargain with yourself that 'it's just this once', you quietly erode your own trust in yourself – your belief that you will actually do what you said you'd do. Your standards are promises you make to yourself. Never break a promise to yourself. Not because you need to be rigid and joyless, but because the self-trust that comes from keeping your own commitments is one of the most valuable things you can build. It's also one of the most powerful forms of self-respect.

4. Stop accepting your own poor excuses

This might sound harsh, but it's honest and it works. The self-trust you build by keeping small commitments to yourself is one of the most valuable things in this process, and you will notice it starts to transfer to other areas of your life. Many of my clients go on to get promotions, change careers, leave unhappy relationships or start the business they have always wanted to start. Sometimes all of that! This is no fluke; the confidence and self-belief you build by developing self-trust, showing up for yourself every day and achieving hard things – like losing fat and actually keeping it off this time – carries forward into the rest of your life.

5. Have the courage to stand out

If you want more from life, you are going to stand out. Most people settle for a mediocre life, and – consciously or not – they want you to do the same. They will comment on your choices, offer opinions on your habits and subtly pull you back towards average with their judgements and their 'you don't want to be obsessed with it' and their 'life's too short to be that strict'. Let them have their opinion; maybe yours is that life is too short to waste your potential and to sit in comfort instead of pushing yourself to see what you could achieve. It's not your job to change their minds or to justify yourself – that is wasted energy. Every time you say no to the easy, default, average choice, you're saying yes to your goals, your values and the life you actually want.

What This Means Day to Day

I want to be clear that the f*ck average mentality isn't about constant intensity. It's not about never resting, never enjoying yourself and never having a night off. That's not average-free living – that's burnout, and burnout is its own kind of average.

F*ck average is about intention, not perfection. It's about the orientation of your choices, not the flawlessness of their execution. It's about noticing when you're drifting and choosing to redirect and live your life intentionally. It's about holding your standard for yourself – not someone else – and showing up for it even when it's inconvenient because you respect yourself enough to show up for yourself when it's hard.

Most days, f*ck average looks incredibly boring from the outside. It looks like eating a high-protein breakfast when you'd rather not think about food yet. Like doing your workout even though the weather is terrible and Netflix is calling. Like going to bed at a reasonable time when the group chat is still going. Like saying no to another glass of wine because you know how you'll feel tomorrow. Like showing up to the thing you said you'd do even though you're tired and nobody would notice if you didn't. (The important thing is that you would notice.) It's not glamorous. It's not a dramatic transformation montage. It's a daily series of small choices that, compounded over months and years, produce a life that looks and feels completely different from the one produced by drift.

Lean into being a bit weird. Allow people to comment on your food choices, the fact that you walk in the rain or that you don't spend every evening watching Netflix. Decide to take responsibility for your life. Stop waiting for someone else to come and do it for you. Decide what you want and go for it.

At 80, you are going to want to have a good story. You are going to want to have taken the risks, tried the things, built the body, shown up for your own life. You are not going to wish you'd blended in more.

F*ck average. F*ck boring social norms. F*ck society's expectations of what you should do and who you should be. Life is too short to do it any other way.

Every time you say no to the easy, default, average choice, you're saying yes to your goals, your values and the life you actually want.

KEY POINTS

- Identity is more durable than motivation. Every consistent action is a vote for the kind of person you are becoming. Given enough time, healthy behaviours stop feeling like discipline and start feeling like simply how you live and become part of who you are.
- F*ck average is a framework, not a demand for perfection. It's about the orientation of your choices and holding high personal standards, not flawless execution.
- Average is not a neutral baseline. It's a specific destination: overweight, tired, stuck. The gap between average and genuinely healthy isn't enormous – the bar is just set low.

- Have the courage to stand out. People will comment. Let them. Every time you choose your goals over the easy option, you're voting for the life you actually want.
- Your environment can be deliberately redesigned: who you spend time with, what food is visible and accessible, what social activities you organise. These changes reduce the willpower required to live differently.
- Going against social norms is uncomfortable. It gets easier. And the life on the other side of that discomfort is worth the temporary friction.

Final Note

This book started with a promise: to tell you the truth about fat loss. And now you know it. The science is not complicated. The marketing around it makes it appear so. Now you know the difference. That is one of the most powerful things I can give you. I hope that you're never conned by confusing fat-loss messaging again.

You've read about energy balance and hunger hormones, about cortisol myths and supplement industry tricks, about the menstrual cycle and menopause and the ageing process. You've read about habits and mindset, range targets, the stories you tell yourself and the power of what you expect. That's a lot of information.

But the frame that underlies all of it is simpler than any of that: health is the best investment you will ever make and, like the best investments, it is simple and it compounds.

The Compound Interest of Your Body

Most people think about health the way they think about spending – you pay for it now and you get the return now. You go to the gym today, you feel better today. You eat well this week, you lose a pound this week. And that's true. But it's only the surface of what's actually happening.

The real return on health compounds. Every workout you complete makes the next one slightly easier. Every week of adequate protein builds a little more muscle. Every good night of sleep improves your cognitive function the next day, which makes better decisions more likely, which makes the next week slightly more consistent. Every year of resistance training builds bone density that protects you from fractures in your seventies. Every decade of healthy habits reduces your risk of type 2 diabetes, cardiovascular disease and dementia.

These returns aren't dramatic or visible day to day. Compound interest never is. But over years and decades, they are enormous. The difference in health, independence and quality of life between a person who has invested consistently in their body and one who hasn't is dramatic. Not just in how they look, but in how they live and the quality of their lives.

The Cost of Not Investing

There's another way to see this. Every time you don't invest – every year of inactivity, every decade of poor sleep, every period of chronic stress left unmanaged, every time you spend a few months out of the gym or let your diet slip for more than a few days – there is a cost. And that cost also compounds.

Sarcopenia – the age-related loss of muscle – accelerates rapidly without resistance training, typically from the fifth decade onwards. Bone density loss, which dramatically increases fracture risk later in life, also accelerates without the loading stress of exercise and adequate calcium and vitamin D. Metabolic health deteriorates when consistently poor food choices and low activity allow body fat to accumulate in places it shouldn't be – the liver and around the organs. Each of these processes feeds the others.

I'm not telling you this to alarm you. I'm telling you because the most important things in life tend not to have a deadline. No one is coming to tell you that you need to get in shape now or that you need to spend more time with your parents now or that you won't always have the energy to go on that holiday and you should book it now or that you should start that business you've always wanted to now. We always think we have more time, we lull ourselves into a false sense of security and say we will start later. But that time often never comes if it's important – so take action now. The earlier you start investing, the greater the compounding return. The later you start, the higher the cost of the catch-up.

If two people both invest £300 per month at an average annual return of 7 per cent, the difference between starting at 20 and starting at 40 is extraordinary. The 20-year-old who invests consistently until age 60 will have contributed £144,000 and ended up with roughly £790,000. The 40-year-old, investing the same £300 per month until 60, will have contributed £72,000 and ended up with around £155,000. The younger investor doesn't just have more because they invested more – they have more because their money had 20 extra years to compound. Time, not intensity, did the heavy lifting. And once those early decades are gone, they cannot be bought back cheaply.

The same is true with your health investment. But look, we don't have time travel, so the earliest you can start is now. And it is never too late to begin. The body is remarkably responsive to investment, at any age. Starting at 50 is better than starting at 55.

Starting at 65 is better than not starting at all. The returns may come more slowly, but they come.

There will always be a reason to wait – for life to be less busy, for the right moment, for more clarity, for the kids to be older, for work to calm down. Opportunities don't wait until you're ready. Live your life as though you're terrified of regret. Because at 80, you are not going to wish you'd played it safer. The far bigger risk is wasting your life waiting for the right time.

Health is Wealth

I chose this heading deliberately. Not because being healthy makes you financially wealthy – although there's decent evidence it's associated with higher earnings, lower healthcare costs and greater productivity. But because health is a form of wealth in the most fundamental sense.

True wealth is not a number in a bank account. It's the capacity to live the life you want. It is freedom. And no amount of money compensates for a body that can't keep up with the life you want to live. The woman who can hike the mountain with her children. Who has the energy to be present at the end of a long week. Who can play on the floor with her grandchildren. Who travels independently in her seventies and eighties. Whose mind stays sharp. Whose mood is broadly stable. Who sleeps well and wakes up feeling capable. That is wealth.

Every healthy habit is a deposit into that account. Every workout, every high-protein meal, every eight hours of sleep, every well-managed stressful period. Small deposits, consistently made over years. The balance grows in ways that aren't always visible – until suddenly, at 55 or 65 or 70, they are very visible indeed. That is when your hard work really comes to fruition. You will be very pleased with how well you looked after yourself.

The Life You're Actually Building Towards

I want you to think about your perfect day. Not the Maldives fantasy; a realistic perfect day for you. The day that shows you living your best, most aligned life. Waking up with energy. Moving your body because you want to, not as punishment. Eating food that genuinely fuels you. Being present with the people you love. Doing work that feels purposeful. Going to bed at the end of it feeling like you lived the day rather than just survived it.

Here's what I've noticed after years of coaching: when women are really honest about what their perfect day looks like, it almost never involves being thinner as the central feature. It involves having energy. It involves confidence. It involves not spending mental bandwidth on food and guilt and what their body looks like. It involves being fully present rather than partially absent because their relationship with their body is taking up too much space in their head.

The fat-loss goal and the rich life goal are not the same goal. But they point in the same direction, and they support each other. Losing excess body fat improves your energy, your mood, your sleep, your mobility, your confidence and your long-term health. Those things make the rich life more accessible. The rich life – the one with genuine connection, purpose, movement you enjoy and food that's enjoyable and flexible – makes sustainable fat loss far easier. The two reinforce each other when you approach them in the right way.

The approach that works is never the one that conflicts with your values. It's never the one that makes you dread mealtimes or resent your social life or feel like you're perpetually waiting to be finished with a diet so you can start living again. That approach produces short-term results and long-term yo-yo cycles, which we already know you want to avoid. The approach that actually works is the one that fits the life you already have and builds towards the life you want. That's what everything in this book has been pointing towards. Fat loss should make your life better, not worse.

What You've Actually Just Done

I want to take a moment here, before we get to the ending, to acknowledge something. If you've read this far, you have done something that most people don't do. Not because most people don't want to feel better or change their bodies – almost everyone does. But because sitting with 28 chapters of information that challenges things you've believed for years, that asks you to think differently about your body and your habits and your relationship with food, is genuinely uncomfortable. It's much easier to buy the supplement, follow the protocol and stay in the familiar cycle.

You didn't do that. You stayed. You read about the hunger hormones and the supplement industry and the misinformation and the mindset. You read the parts that probably made you think about previous attempts and feel something complicated about them. You're still here.

That matters. Not as a small motivational pat on the back – it actually matters, practically, for your results. Because the biggest predictor of long-term success isn't the quality of your meal plan. It's whether you understand why you're doing what you're doing. Whether the approach makes sense to you at a level deeper than 'I was told to'. You now understand why. That's a different starting point from every previous attempt, and it changes what's possible.

What This Book Was Actually About

The surface of this book is about fat loss. But fat loss was always just the entry point. What this book is actually about is giving you the understanding and the tools to build a body and a life that supports everything you want to do in it – for as long as possible, as well as possible.

Fat loss, approached with the right understanding, is not a punishment or a restriction. It's one part of that investment in your health and quality of life. Reducing excess body fat – particularly visceral fat around the organs – reduces inflammation, improves insulin sensitivity, lowers cardiovascular risk, reduces joint load and improves sleep. It's one of the most powerful health interventions available to most people, and it's largely within your control.

But it only works that way when it's part of a bigger picture. When it's built on genuine food knowledge rather than fear and restriction. When it's supported by sleep, stress management and strength training. When the goal is long-term health, energy and function rather than a number on the scales by a specific date. When it's sustainable, evidence-based and kind – to your body and to yourself.

I want to end with something I say to almost every client I work with, usually somewhere in the first few sessions: you are not broken. Your body is not working against you. You are not uniquely difficult, hormonally chaotic or metabolically disadvantaged. You are a person with a completely normal body responding to physiology and behaviour in entirely predictable ways. And predictable means manageable.

You don't need the supplement that 'finally understands women's bodies'. You don't need to wait until life gets less busy or until you feel ready or until you've sorted everything else out first. You don't need a specialist protocol because you're over 40 or perimenopausal. You don't need to have it all figured out before you start.

You need the right information – which you now have. You need a strategy that fits your actual life – which this book has given you the tools to build. And you need to believe, with genuine conviction, that change is possible. Because it is. Completely. For everyone. I have never worked with a woman whose body was incapable of change. Not once. The women who don't change are the ones who never quite believe they can, and so never quite fully try. Don't be that woman. You've read too much to still believe the story that your body is the problem. And you don't need to believe you can lose all the weight you need to or that you can run a marathon. You need to believe you can set some realistic range targets that will push you in the direction of your goals and stick to them. For one week. Just one week. That is all you need to build momentum.

I want you to use what you've learned in this book for the rest of your life. Please don't just sit on this information and let it become another book you've read and not implemented. Action it. Start now. It's not going to get easier or less busy. Set yourself some range targets, ones that are in line with your goals and start. And if you need my help, head to my website where you can message me – I reply to every single one. Whatever you do, don't do nothing.

Where to Find Me

Writing this book has been one of the most satisfying things I've done professionally, and that's largely because of the women I've had the privilege of working with and learning from over the years. Every client who came in convinced she was broken and left knowing she wasn't has shaped how I think about this work and how I try to communicate it.

If you want to continue the conversation, the podcast is the best place to start. I cover new research, answer questions and work through specific topics that don't fit neatly into a book. It's free, it's honest, and it's very anti bullsh*t and real. Look up the *ESGfitness* podcast wherever you get yours.

If you want more structured support – whether that's working with me directly or finding the right coach for where you are right now – the website is esgfitness.co.uk. Coaching isn't right for everyone at every stage, but if you've been trying to do this alone for a while and you're not getting the results you want, it's worth considering. The right support doesn't just speed things up – it changes what feels possible.

And if this book helped you – if something in it shifted the way you think about your body or your approach or yourself – I'd genuinely love to know. The best thing you can do for someone who wrote something is tell them it landed. That, and lend it to someone who might benefit too!

Finally, I want to sincerely thank you for your attention and time. That is a huge gift and I am truly honoured you've given me so much of it. I hope it has been worth it.

Appendix: Protein in Common Foods

All figures are approximate and based on typical cooked weights, unless otherwise stated. Protein content varies slightly by brand, cooking method and cut. Use this as a working guide, not an exact science – consistency matters far more than precision.

FOOD	TYPICAL PORTION	PROTEIN (APPROX.)
Meat & Poultry		
Chicken breast, cooked	1 medium (150g)	~45g
Turkey breast, cooked	1 medium slice (150g)	~44g
Lean beef mince, cooked	150g	~36g
Sirloin steak, cooked	150g	~38g
Pork loin, cooked	150g	~37g
Back bacon, grilled	2 rashers (60g)	~14g
Fish & Seafood		
Tuna, tinned in water (drained)	1 standard tin (145g)	~34g
Salmon fillet, cooked	1 fillet (150g)	~30g

APPENDIX: PROTEIN IN COMMON FOODS

FOOD	TYPICAL PORTION	PROTEIN (APPROX.)
Cod fillet, cooked	1 fillet (150g)	~26g
Mackerel fillet, cooked	1 fillet (130g)	~25g
Sardines, tinned in brine	1 tin (100g)	~24g
King prawns, cooked	150g	~29g
Smoked salmon	100g	~20g
Eggs & Dairy		
Eggs, large	2 eggs	~12g
Greek yoghurt (full-fat)	200g pot	~20g
Skyr / Icelandic yoghurt	150g pot	~14g
Cottage cheese	200g	~24g
Quark	200g	~22g
Cheddar cheese	1 matchbox portion (30g)	~8g
Milk, semi-skimmed	1 glass (250ml)	~9g
Plant-Based Proteins		
Tofu, firm	150g	~18g
Tempeh	100g	~19g
Edamame (shelled)	150g	~18g
Lentils, cooked	200g	~18g
Chickpeas, cooked	200g	~16g
Kidney beans / black beans, cooked	200g	~15g
Soya mince, cooked	100g	~17g
Convenient & Snack Sources		
Whey protein shake	1 scoop (30g) + water	~22–25g
Protein bar	1 bar (60g)	~20g

FOOD	TYPICAL PORTION	PROTEIN (APPROX.)
Protein yoghurt	1 pot (200g)	~20g
Peanut butter	2 tbsp (30g)	~8g
Almonds	Small handful (30g)	~6g
Oats (dry)	1 serving (50g)	~5g
Quinoa, cooked	200g	~8g
Edamame snack pack	1 pack (90g)	~11g

A reminder: you're aiming for roughly 1.6–2.2g of protein per kilogram of your body weight per day. For most women, that means building a meaningful source of protein into every meal – not sprinkling a little on top.

References

CHAPTER 1 THE SCIENCE OF FAT LOSS

Meerman, R. and Brown, A. J., 'When somebody loses weight, where does the fat go?', *The BMJ* 349 (2014), g7257.

CHAPTER 2 WHY FAT LOSS IS HARDER FOR WOMEN (AND WHY THAT'S NOT AN EXCUSE)

Crescent B. Martin, et al., 'Attempts to Lose Weight Among Adults in the United States, 2013–2016', *NCHS Data Brief 313, National Center for Health Statistics* (2018).

Pillitteri, J., et al., 'Use of dietary supplements for weight loss in the United States: results of a national survey', *Obesity* 16:4 (2008), pp. 790–6.

Prevos, P., 'Difference between male and female body image statistics', horizonofreason.com (2005).

Gualdi-Russo, E., et al., 'Sex differences in body image perception and ideals: Analysis of possible determinants', *International Journal of Environmental Research and Public Heal*th 19:5 (2026), p. 2745.

Voges, M.M., et al., 'Gender differences in body evaluation: Do men show more self-serving double standards than women?', *Frontiers in Psychology* 10 (2019).

Weeks, A.C. and Ruppanner, L., 'A typology of US parents' mental loads: Core and episodic cognitive labor', *Journal of Marriage and Family* 87:3 (2025), pp. 966–89.

CHAPTER 3 WHY FAT LOSS FEELS SO COMPLICATED

Johnston, B.C., et al., 'Comparison of weight loss among named diet programs in overweight and obese adults: a meta-analysis', *Journal of the American Medical Association* 312:9 (2014), pp. 923–33.

CHAPTER 5 SETTING UP YOUR FAT-LOSS CALORIES IN A WAY THAT ACTUALLY WORKS

Westenhoefer, J., et al., 'Validation of the flexible and rigid control dimensions of dietary restraint', *International Journal of Eating Disorders* 26:1 (1999), pp. 53–64.

CHAPTER 7 THE STARVATION MODE MYTH

Stewart, W.K. and Fleming, L.W., 'Features of a successful therapeutic fast of 382 days' duration', *Postgraduate Medical Journal* 49:569 (1973), pp. 203–9.

CHAPTER 8 THE CORTISOL CON

Tomiyama, A.J., et al., 'Low calorie dieting increases cortisol', *Psychosomatic Medicine* 72:4 (2010), pp. 357–64.

Caplin, A., et al., 'The effects of exercise intensity on the cortisol response to a subsequent acute psychosocial stressor', *Psychoneuroendocrinology* 131:105336 (2021).

Childs, E. and de Wit, H., 'Regular exercise is associated with emotional resilience to acute stress in healthy adults', *Frontiers in Physiology* 5:161 (2014).

De Nys, L., et al., 'The effects of physical activity on cortisol and sleep: a systematic review and meta-analysis', *Psychoneuroendocrinology* 143:105843 (2022).

Hunter, M.R., et al., 'Urban nature experiences reduce stress in the context of daily life based on salivary biomarkers', *Frontiers in Psychology* 10:722 (2019).

Stephens, M.A. and Wand, G., 'Stress and the HPA axis: role of glucocorticoids in alcohol dependence', *Alcohol Research* 34:4 (2012), pp. 468–83.

Uchino, B.N., 'Social support and health: a review of physiological processes potentially underlying links to disease outcomes', *Journal of Behavioral Medicine* 29:4 (2006), pp. 377–87.

CHAPTER 9 THE GLUCOSE OBSESSION

Hall, K.D., et al., 'Energy expenditure and body composition changes after an isocaloric ketogenic diet in overweight and obese men', *American Journal of Clinical Nutrition* 104:2 (2016), pp. 324–33.

CHAPTER 10 DON'T BUY ANOTHER SUPPLEMENT UNTIL YOU'VE READ THIS

Myung, S.K. and Park, Y., 'Effects of collagen supplements on skin aging: a systematic review and meta-analysis of randomized controlled trials', *American Journal of Medicine* 138:9 (2025), pp. 1264–77.

Oikawa S.Y., et al., 'Whey protein but not collagen peptides stimulate acute and longer-term muscle protein synthesis with and without resistance exercise in healthy older women: a randomized controlled trial', *American Journal of Clinical Nutrition* 111:3 (2020), pp. 708–18.

Choi, F.D., et al., 'Oral collagen supplementation: a systematic review of dermatological applications', *Journal of Drugs in Dermatology* 18:1 (2019), pp. 9–16.

Ravindran, R., 'Collagen supplementation for skin and musculoskeletal health: An umbrella review of meta-analyses on elasticity, hydration, and structural outcomes', *Aesthetic Surgery Journal Open Forum* Vol. 8 (2026).

Chiou, W.B., Yang, C.C. and Wan, C.S., 'Ironic effects of dietary supplementation: illusory invulnerability created by taking dietary supplements licenses health-risk behaviors', *Psychological Science* 22:8 (2011), pp. 1081–6.

Cohen, P.A., et al., 'Presence and quantity of botanical ingredients with purported performance-enhancing properties in sports supplements', *JAMA Network Open* 6:7 (2023), e2323879.

Zmora, N., et al., 'Personalized gut mucosal colonization resistance to empiric probiotics is associated with unique host and microbiome features', *Cell* 174:6 (2018), pp. 1388–1405.

Lopresti, A.L., Smith, S.J., Malvi, H. and Kodgule, R., 'An investigation into the stress-relieving and pharmacological actions of an ashwagandha (Withania somnifera) extract: A randomized, double-blind, placebo-controlled study', *Medicine* 98:37 (2019), e17186.

Dulloo, A.G., et al., 'Efficacy of a green tea extract rich in catechin polyphenols and caffeine in increasing 24-h energy expenditure and fat oxidation in humans', *American Journal of Clinical Nutrition* 70:6 (1999), pp. 1040–5.

Wilding, J.P.H., et al., 'Once-weekly semaglutide in adults with overweight or obesity', *New England Journal of Medicine* 384:11 (2021).

Hollis, B.W. and Wagner, C.L., 'Clinical review: The role of the parent compound vitamin D with respect to metabolism and function:

Why clinical dose intervals can affect clinical outcomes', *Journal of Clinical Endocrinology and Metabolism* 96:9 (2011), pp. 2563–72. Multiple researchers and bodies (including the Endocrine Society) recommend 1,500–2,000 IU daily for at-risk groups.

Mozaffarian D. and Wu, J.H.Y., 'Omega-3 fatty acids and cardiovascular disease: effects on risk factors, molecular pathways, and clinical events', *Journal of the American College of Cardiology* 58:20 (2011), pp. 2047–67.

Kreider R.B., et al., 'International Society of Sports Nutrition position stand: safety and efficacy of creatine supplementation in exercise, sport, and medicine', *Journal of International Society of Sports Nutrition* 14:18 (2017).

Vandenberghe K., et al., 'Long-term creatine intake is beneficial to muscle performance during resistance training', *Journal of Applied Physiology* 83:6 (1997), pp. 2055–63.

Chilibeck, P.D., et al., 'Effect of creatine supplementation during resistance training on lean tissue mass and muscular strength in older adults: a meta-analysis', *Open Access Journal of Sports Medicine* 8 (2017), pp. 213–26.

CHAPTER 11 MOOD FIRST

Achor, S., *The Happiness Advantage* (Crown Business, 2010). The core research the book draws on includes Fredrickson's broaden-and-build theory: Fredrickson, B.L., 'The role of positive emotions in positive psychology', *American Psychologist* 56:3 (2001), pp. 218–26.

Seligman M.E.P., et al., 'Positive psychology progress: empirical validation of interventions', *American Psychologist* 60:5 (2005), pp. 410–21.

Kahneman D. and Snell J., 'Predicting a changing taste: do people know what they will like?', *Journal of Behavioral Decision Making* 5:3 (1992), pp. 187–200.

Tuk, M.A., et al., 'Better moods for better eating? How mood influences food choice', *Journal of Consumer Psychology* 25:1 (2015), pp. 111–22.

Garg, N., Wansink, B. and Inman, J.J., 'The influence of incidental affect on consumers' food intake', *Journal of Marketing* 71:1 (2007), pp. 194–206.

Monteiro, C.A., et al., 'Ultra-processed foods: what they are and how to identify them', *Public Health Nutrition* 22:5 (2019), pp. 936–41. For UPF consumption and mental health: Adjibade, M., et al., 'Prospective association between ultra-processed food consumption and incident depressive symptoms', *JAMA Internal Medicine* 179:10 (2019), pp. 1373–80.

CHAPTER 12 THE STORY YOU TELL YOURSELF

Crum, A.J., Corbin, W.R., Brownell, K.D. and Salovey, P., 'Mind over milkshakes: Mindsets, not just nutrients, determine ghrelin response', *Health Psychology* 30:4 (2011), pp. 424–9.

Foad, A.J., et al., 'Pharmacological and psychological effects of caffeine on cycling time trial performance', *Medicine and Science in Sports and Exercise* 40:12 (2008), pp. 2109–16.

Crum, A.J., Salovey, P. and Achor, S., 'Rethinking stress: The role of mindsets in determining the stress response', *Journal of Personality and Social Psychology* 104:4 (2013), pp. 716–33.

CHAPTER 13 THE EXPECTATION EFFECT

Crum, A.J., Corbin, W.R., Brownell, K.D. and Salovey, P., 'Mind over milkshakes: Mindsets, not just nutrients, determine ghrelin response', *Health Psychology* 30:4 (2011), pp. 424–90.

Crum, A.J. and Langer, E.J., 'Mind-set matters: Exercise and the placebo effect', *Psychological Science* 18:2 (2007), pp. 165–71.

REFERENCES

CHAPTER 14 START WITH ENERGY

Hood, D.A., et al., 'Maintenance of skeletal muscle mitochondria in health, exercise, and aging', *Annual Review of Physiology* 81 (2019), pp.19–41.

CHAPTER 15 DECIDE ONCE

VanEpps, E.M., Downs, J.S. and Loewenstein, G., 'Advance ordering for healthier eating? Field experiments on the relationship between the meal order–consumption time delay and meal content', *Journal of Marketing Research* 53:3 (2016), pp. 369–80.

Nawijn, J., et al., 'Vacationers happier, but most not happier after a holiday', *Applied Research in Quality of Life* 5:1 (2010), pp. 35–47.

Chun, H.H., Diehl, K. and MacInnis, D.J., 'Savoring an upcoming experience affects ongoing and remembered consumption enjoyment', *Journal of Marketing* 81:3 (2017), pp. 96–110.

Loewenstein, G., 'Anticipation and the valuation of delayed consumption', *Economic Journal* 97:387 (1987), pp. 666–84.

Christensen, C.M., 'How Will You Measure Your Life? (extract)', *Working Knowledge*, Harvard Business School (2012).

Baumeister, R.F., Bratslavsky, E., Muraven, M. and Tice, D.M., 'Ego depletion: Is the active self a limited resource?', *Journal of Personality and Social Psychology* 74:5 (1998), pp. 1252–65.

Danziger, S., et al., 'Extraneous factors in judicial decisions', *Proceedings of the National Academy of Sciences* 108:17 (2011), pp. 6889–92.

Clear, J., *Atomic Habits: An Easy and Proven Way to Build Good Habits and Break Bad Ones* (Avery/Penguin Random House, 2018).

CHAPTER 16 MAKING YOUR BAD DAYS LESS BAD

Gollwitzer, P.M. and Sheeran, P., 'Implementation intentions and goal achievement: a meta-analysis of effects and processes', *Advances in Experimental Social Psychology* 38 (2006), pp. 69–119.

CHAPTER 17 PROTEIN: THE ONE THING THAT ACTUALLY EARNS ITS PLACE

Morton, R.W., et al., 'A systematic review, meta-analysis and meta-regression of the effect of protein supplementation on resistance training-induced gains in muscle mass and strength', *British Journal of Sports Medicine* 52:6 (2018), pp. 376–84.

CHAPTER 18 THE 3:1 METHOD

Aune, D., et al., 'Fruit and vegetable intake and the risk of cardiovascular disease, total cancer and all-cause mortality', *International Journal of Epidemiology* 46:3 (2017), pp.1029–56.

CHAPTER 19 EXERCISE: THE MAGIC PILL

Barry V.W., et al., 'Fitness vs. fatness on all-cause mortality: a meta-analysis', *Progress in Cardiovascular Diseases* 56:4 (2014), pp. 382–90.

Levine, J.A., 'Non-exercise activity thermogenesis (NEAT)', *Best Practice and Research: Clinical Endocrinology and Metabolism* 16:4 (2002), pp. 679–702.

Noetel, M., et al., 'Effect of exercise for depression: systematic review and network meta-analysis of randomised controlled trials', *The BMJ* 384 (2024), e075847.

CHAPTER 20 SLEEP: THE FAT-LOSS TOOL YOU'RE IGNORING

Spiegel, K., et al., 'Sleep curtailment in healthy young men is associated with decreased leptin levels, elevated ghrelin levels, and increased hunger and appetite', *Annals of Internal Medicine* 141:11 (2004), pp. 846–50.

Greer, S.M., et al., 'The impact of sleep deprivation on food desire in the human brain', *Nature Communications* 4 (2013), p. 2259.

Hanlon, E.C., et al., 'Sleep restriction enhances the daily rhythm of circulating levels of endocannabinoid 2-arachidonoylglycerol', *Sleep* 39:3 (2016), pp. 653–64.

St-Onge, M.P., et al., 'Sleep restriction leads to increased activation of brain regions sensitive to food stimuli', *American Journal of Clinical Nutrition* 95:4 (2012), pp. 818–24.

Tasali, E., et al., 'Effect of sleep extension on objectively assessed energy intake among adults with overweight', *Journal of the American Medical Association: Internal Medicine* 182:4 (2022), pp. 365–74.

Nedeltcheva, A.V., et al., 'Insufficient sleep undermines dietary efforts to reduce adiposity', *Annals of Internal Medicine* 153:7 (2010), pp. 435–41.

Walker, M., *Why We Sleep* (Scribner, 2017). Also: Van Cauter, E., et al., 'Metabolic consequences of sleep and sleep loss', *Sleep Medicine* 9:Suppl. 1 (2008), pp. S23–8.

Irwin, M.R., 'Why sleep is important for health: a psychoneuroimmunology perspective', *Annual Review of Psychology* 66 (2015), pp. 143–72.

CHAPTER 21 THE ULTIMATE GUIDE TO REDUCING HUNGER: 13 FACTORS YOU HAVEN'T CONSIDERED

Stelmach-Mardas, M., et al., 'Link between food energy density and body weight changes in obese adults', *Nutrients* 8:4 (2016), p. 229.

Rolls, B.J., 'The relationship between dietary energy density and energy intake', *Physiology and Behavior* 97:5 (2009), pp. 609–15.

Howarth, N.C., Saltzman, E. and Roberts, S.B., 'Dietary fiber and energy regulation', *Nutrition Reviews* 59:5 (2001), pp. 129–39.

DiMeglio, D.P. and Mattes, R.D., 'Liquid versus solid carbohydrate: effects on food intake and body weight', *International Journal of Obesity* 24:6 (2000), pp. 794–800.

Baumeister, R.F., Bratslavsky, E., Muraven, M. and Tice, D.M., 'Ego depletion: Is the active self a limited resource?', *Journal of Personality and Social Psychology* 74:5 (1998), pp. 1252–65.

Privitera, G.J. and Creary, H.E., 'Proximity and visibility of fruits and vegetables influence intake in a kitchen setting among college students', *Environment and Behavior* 45:7 (2013), pp. 876–86.

Rolls, B.J., 'The relationship between dietary energy density and energy intake', *Physiology and Behavior* 97:5 (2009), pp. 609–15.

Lopez, R.B., et al., 'Bottomless bowls revisited: a pre-registered replication and extension', *Journal of Experimental Psychology: General* 153:2 (2024), pp. 275–81.

CHAPTER 22 F*CK YES OR NO

Manson, M., 'Fuck Yes or No', markmanson.net (2013).

Robinson, E., et al., 'A systematic review and meta-analysis examining the effect of eating rate on energy intake and hunger', *American Journal of Clinical Nutrition* 109:3 (2019), pp. 613–28.

de Castro, J.M., 'Family and friends produce greater meal intake than other companions', *Physiology and Behavior* 56:3 (1994), pp. 445–55.

CHAPTER 23 THE MONTHLY SABOTAGE

Hallam, J., et al., 'Gender-related differences in food craving and obesity', *Yale Journal of Biology and Medicine* 92:1 (2019), pp. 101–8.

McNulty, K.L., et al., 'The effects of menstrual cycle phase on exercise performance in eumenorrheic women: a systematic review and meta-analysis', *Sports Medicine* 50 (2020), pp. 1813–27.

CHAPTER 24 THE MENOPAUSE MARKETING CON

Maturana, M.A., et al., 'High-intensity interval training (HIIT) benefits in peri- and postmenopausal women: a systematic review', *Clinical and Experimental Obstetrics and Gynecology* 48:2 (2021), pp. 295–303.

Berin, E., et al., 'Resistance training for hot flushes in postmenopausal women', *Maturitas* 126 (2019), pp. 55–60. Also: Lopez, P., et al., 'Resistance training effectiveness on body composition and body weight outcomes in individuals with overweight and obesity across the lifespan', *Obesity Reviews* 23:5 (2022), e13428.

Manson, J.E. and Kaunitz, A.M., 'Menopause management – getting clinical care back on track', *New England Journal of Medicine* 374:9 (2016), pp. 803–6.

The British Menopause Society (2020) recommends HRT for most women under 60 with significant symptoms, with evidence that benefits outweigh risks in this group.

CHAPTER 25 HOW TO AGE WELL

Daly, L.S., Van Hooren, B. and Jakeman, P., 'Physiological characteristics of a 92-yr-old four-time world champion indoor rower', *Journal of Applied Physiology* 135:6 (2023), pp. 1415–20.

Pontzer, H., et al., 'Daily energy expenditure through the human life course', *Science* 373:6556 (2021), pp. 808–12.

Howe, T.E., et al., 'Exercise for preventing and treating osteoporosis in postmenopausal women', *Cochrane Database of Systematic Reviews* 7 (2011), CD000333.

CHAPTER 26 WHY MAINTENANCE MATTERS

Mann, T., et al., 'Medicare's search for effective obesity treatments: Diets are not the answer', *American Psychologist* 62:3 (2007), pp. 220–33.

Wing, R.R. and Phelan, S., 'Long-term weight loss maintenance', *American Journal of Clinical Nutrition* 82:1 (2005), 222S–225S.

Thomas, J.G., et al., 'Weight-loss maintenance for 10 years in the

National Weight Control Registry', *American Journal of Preventive Medicine* 46:1 (2014), pp. 17–23.

Knowler, W.C., et al., 'Reduction in the incidence of type 2 diabetes with lifestyle intervention or metformin', *New England Journal of Medicine* 346:6 (2022), pp. 393–403.

Gregg, E.W., et al., 'Association of the magnitude of weight loss and changes in physical fitness with long-term cardiovascular disease outcomes in overweight or obese people with type 2 diabetes: a post-hoc analysis of the Look AHEAD randomised clinical trial', *The Lancet Diabetes and Endocrinology* 4:11 (2016), pp. 913–21.

Chlebowski, R.T., et al., 'Weight loss and breast cancer incidence in postmenopausal women', *Journal of Clinical Oncology* 37:31 (2019), pp. 2839–47.

Mackie, G.M., Samocha-Bonet, D. and Tam, C.S., 'Does weight cycling promote obesity and metabolic risk factors?', *Obesity Research and Clinical Practice* 11:2 (2017), pp. 131–9.

CHAPTER 27 WHAT PEOPLE WHO SUCCESSFULLY MAINTAIN ACTUALLY DO

Thomas, J.G., et al., 'Weight-loss maintenance for 10 years in the National Weight Control Registry', *American Journal of Preventive Medicine* 46:1 (2014), pp. 17–23.

Peterson, N.D., et al., 'Dietary self-monitoring and long-term success with weight management', *Obesity* 22:9 (2014), pp. 1962–7.

CHAPTER 28 F*CK AVERAGE: THE MAINTENANCE MINDSET

Herman, C.P. and Polivy, J., 'The self-regulation of eating: theoretical and practical problems' in R.F. Baumeister and K.D. Vohs (eds.), *Handbook of Self-Regulation* (The Guilford Press, 2004).

REFERENCES

Robinson, E., et al., 'What everyone else is eating: a systematic review and meta-analysis of the effect of informational eating norms on eating behavior', *Journal of the Academy of Nutrition and Dietetics* 114:3 (2014), pp. 414–29.

FINAL NOTE

Lim, S.S., et al., 'A comparative risk assessment of burden of disease', *The Lancet* 380:9859 (2012), pp. 2224–60. For health and financial wellbeing: Oswald, A.J. and Powdthavee, N., 'Does happiness adapt?', *Journal of Public Economics* 92:5–6 (2008), pp. 1061–77.

With Thanks

To my parents – for everything that came before this book. You gave me the belief that I was capable of hard things before I had any evidence that was true. You taught me to question everything and always think for myself. You've supported me unconditionally and always pushed me to achieve more. I'm so grateful for your unwavering love and support.

To my friends for always making the hard days easier and celebrating my wins louder than I do. Special mention to Emilia, Courtney, Kate, Katie and Chloe for way too many pep-talk voice notes.

To Molly – you are incredibly kind, endlessly supportive and very, very patient. You are my constant source of motivation. Thank you. I love you.

To my wonderful editors – Julia and Sam – for believing in the book and seeing potential before there was proof. I came in with a message I believed in. You helped me find the words to communicate it.

And the biggest thanks to every client who has ever trusted me with their goals, their frustrations, their spirals and their wins – this book is for you and it is as much yours as it is mine. You taught me everything I know about what actually works in real life. I hope you see yourselves in these pages, and I hope you're proud of how far you've come. And I hope I have done you proud with this book.

Index

Note: pages numbers in **bold** refer to diagrams, pages numbers in italics refer to information contained in tables.

INDEX

INDEX

INDEX

INDEX

INDEX

INDEX